Connected Objects in Health

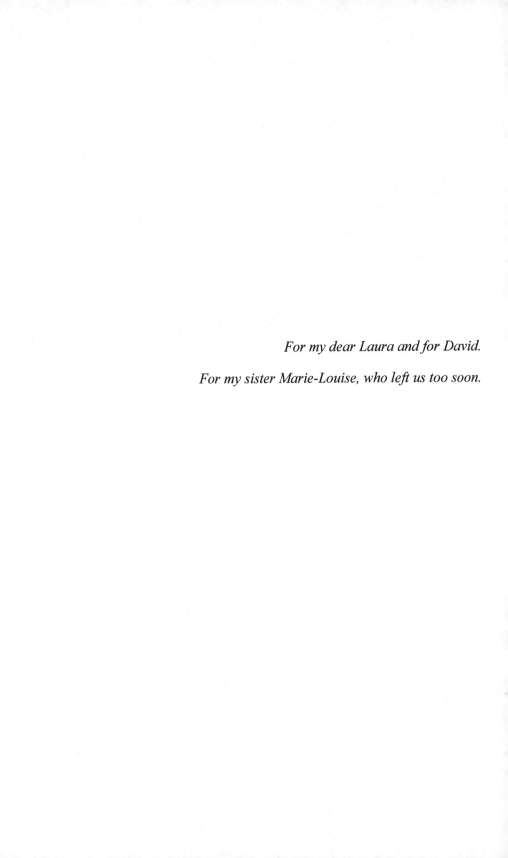

For my dear Laura and for David.

For my sister Marie-Louise, who left us too soon.

Health Industrialization Set

coordinated by
Bruno Salgues

Connected Objects in Health

Risks, Uses and Perspectives

Laure Beyala

First published 2017 in Great Britain and the United States by ISTE Press Ltd and Elsevier Ltd

ISTE Press Ltd
27-37 St George's Road
London SW19 4EU
UK

www.iste.co.uk

Elsevier Ltd
The Boulevard, Langford Lane
Kidlington, Oxford, OX5 1GB
UK

www.elsevier.com

Notices

Knowledge and best practice in this field are constantly changing. As new research and experience broaden our understanding, changes in research methods, professional practices, or medical treatment may become necessary.

Practitioners and researchers must always rely on their own experience and knowledge in evaluating and using any information, methods, compounds, or experiments described herein. In using such information or methods they should be mindful of their own safety and the safety of others, including parties for whom they have a professional responsibility.

To the fullest extent of the law, neither the Publisher nor the authors, contributors, or editors, assume any liability for any injury and/or damage to persons or property as a matter of products liability, negligence or otherwise, or from any use or operation of any methods, products, instructions, or ideas contained in the material herein.

For information on all our publications visit our website at http://store.elsevier.com/

British Library Cataloguing-in-Publication Data
A CIP record for this book is available from the British Library
Library of Congress Cataloging in Publication Data
A catalog record for this book is available from the Library of Congress
ISBN 978-1-78548-259-5

Printed and bound in the UK and US

Contents

Foreword

The connected health revolution, initiated in the wake of the quantified self movement and the mass distribution of smartphones, is profoundly changing our relationship to the body and disease.

This revolution is stimulated in a singular way by private actors in the domain of new technologies: major actors such as Google, Apple, Microsoft and Samsung, just to mention a few, but also a multitude of start-ups that impose their rhythm on the rest of the world.

Despite the significant expectations that it can bring about concerning the reduction of costs, prevention, and telemedicine, connected health must still show what it can do with regard to its real efficacy as well as its ability to spread without calling into question the ethics of medical care.

The rapid emergence of new technologies, and the new healthcare models that they impose, too often cause legislators and actors from civil society to lag behind in analyzing the technological and human risks of this shift.

In my opinion, it is the purpose of books like this present volume to take the time to analyze the different aspects of this connected revolution with tools adapted to this endeavor.

The rigor of the analysis and the breadth of the subject dealt with make this an indispensible book for all who wish to further reflect on this topic.

Benjamin PITRAT

Acknowledgements

At the end of this project, I am convinced that publishing a work is far from an individual task. I could never have completed this book without the support of a large number of people whose generosity, good spirits and interest shown on my behalf allowed me to achieve my goals.

I want to thank:

– Dr. Benjamin Pitrat for having accepted to spontaneously write the foreword to my book;

– the whole team from the ISTE Publishing for their trust;

– my parents and my friends, who supported me throughout the entire process;

– Dr. Vincent Leroux, Alain Desroches and Dr. François Teboul for their valuable advice and their human qualities of listening and understanding.

Introduction

A connected object is made up of sensors that transmit information via a mobile application or an online service. This allows personal data to be recovered to better follow its health indicators so as to monitor their evolution. It also constitutes a support in preventing certain diseases. With the rise of these innovative technologies, connected health is henceforth part of our daily lives and it has today become a subject of great hope.

A new practice has appeared to improve our life habits (health and human well-being): the "quantified self". This is a phenomenon that involves taking one's own health indicators and sharing these data using new information and communication technologies. The processing of these data belongs to the so-called "big data" system.

This phenomenon is powered by the emergence of objects connected to a smartphone, computer or tablet via the Internet, wireless connections such as blood pressure monitors, pedometers, watches, connected medical devices that measure heart rate, devices that allow a person's temperature to be taken precisely and remotely, and many others.

These connected medical devices will transform the users' experience as well as the care pathway, from entering the hospital to returning home. To be efficient, this system, which multiplies the capacities for data analysis, cross-referencing, visualization and sharing, is today a significant scientific progress factor that still has many challenges to overcome, particularly in matters of data security, availability, integrity, confidentiality and interoperability. The European General Data Protection Regulation proposes that data concerning health be defined as "personal data related to the physical or mental health of a natural person, including the provision of health care services, which reveal information about his or her health status"[1].

To manage the risks linked to the use of these connected medical devices, we performed a risk cartography related to the use of connected non-contact thermometers put on the market by certain start-ups. These allow a person's temperature to be taken remotely and this measurement to be instantly transferred to a mobile application via radio waves. We will also focus our attention on the advantages that these kinds of devices could provide to our existential system. This example will serve as a common thread for this work, the concepts and methods of which can be applied to most Internet of Things medical devices.

---

1 Source: http://www.privacy-regulation.eu/en/4.htm.

PART 1

Basic Concepts

Connected Objects

1.1. What is a connected object?

Numerous statistic studies attest to an explosion of connected objects in the world by 2020. According to the Verizon company, the world will contain 25.6 billion connected objects in 2019; between 2014 and 2021, their numbers will triple, going from 9.9 to 30 billion. However, continued vigilance is necessary when reading these numbers. In fact, the very notion of the Internet of Things (IoT), subject to a multitude of interpretations, remains to be defined.

The term "Internet" usually does not extend past the electronic world; the IoT represents the exchanges of information and data from devices present in the real world to Internet servers. It assumes its universal character to designate objects connected to various uses and services.

DEFINITION.– *A connected object is generally defined based on the following five principles:*

– identification: by type or entity (barcode, IP address, etc.);

– sensitivity, for every object is apt for communicating information about its surroundings;

– interactivity: certain objects can only be activated upon exchanging information, while others can be connected permanently or when a connection becomes available;

– a virtual presence through a program that can act on behalf of a physical object to which it is attached and of which it has full knowledge;

– and finally, autonomy: each object is autonomous and independent (it can interact with other objects on the network).

A connected object is visible on the Internet, directly (being connected to it), or indirectly (via equipment). In order to connect a connected object like a blood pressure monitor or a pedometer, for instance, it would be necessary to possess the seven following components:

– a label or a miniature electronic sensor allowing objects to be identified (RFID1, graphic or virtual labels);

– a means of reading the labels;

– a mobile terminal; very often, this is a smartphone, a tablet, a smartwatch. Desktop computers are used at this stage;

– an application or software for the mobile device;

– an IP address or wireless network to transfer or read data (3G[1], Wi-fi, RFID, Bluetooth);

– content, "the temperature for our case study", blood pressure, heart rate, etc.;

– a display screen (LCD[2] or otherwise).

Most often, there is coupled use of a sensor (integrated in a connected object like a watch, for example) and an application (online or mobile).

The IoT thus refers to a whole set allowing the users' data to be captured, recovered, stored, processed and transferred between the virtual and physical worlds without interruption.

Each innovation is accompanied by new uses. Connected objects and applications, in particular, offer us services such as self-evaluation, physical and athletic preparation, satellite or Internet positioning and improved behavior management.

As for health: the assistance with diagnosis and advice, which generates better healthcare.

---

1 "3G" refers to the third generation of mobile phone technologies.
2 A liquid–crystal display (LCD) uses a digital display method on a flat screen.

One thing is certain: if the 1990s were marked by the Internet revolution, the 2000s will forever be those of connected objects. On the market, they are classed by domain: connected objects for health (cardiometer, blood pressure monitor, thermometer, balance, etc.), sports and well-being (in this branch, we find connected FITBIT bracelets[3] that measure the number of steps, heartbeats and sleep), household products (smoke detector, door sensor, alarm, etc.), electrical appliances (connected cat bed, remote for pets, etc.), communication and accessories (connected watch, ring, bracelet, glasses, etc.), childcare and intelligent cities.

1.2. The different categories of connected objects

Given the diversity of the solutions brought by these connected objects, they are grouped into two large categories.

1.2.1. Connected objects having the status of connected medical devices

These connected objects, with the status of connected medical devices, work on three levels:

– they measure an individual's health indicators. It is in this way that they allow a person's physical data to be collected. These data are beneficial:

- for healthcare professionals. They provide more information about the health situation of the patient for the provision of better care;

- for patients, by allowing them to better understand the functioning of their body. They can thereby better cope with a chronic disease. The company Boltgroup, based in North Carolina, has developed a connected watch, "Sugar". This is a connected health device to better follow type 1 and 2 diabetes;

- for in-depth studies on rare pathologies. In fact, they also constitute a gold mine for medical research centers; scientific research requires the statistical analysis of available megadata over a long period of time.

---

3 Original source: http://www.rtl.be/info/magazine/hi-tech/on-a-essaye-le-dernier-fitbit-a-quoi-ca-sert-un-bracelet-connecte–708385.aspx.

– they analyze physical parameters through decisional algorithms integrated into applications. These are installed in the mobile terminal and they circulate information (reminders, warnings, recommendations, etc.) about the user (the patient);

– they act on the individual by allowing him or her to be an actor in the healthcare process or when overcoming a handicap. Itens, for example, develops connected objects allowing chronic pain to be eased.

In France, these are devices that respond to European norms (CE)[4] and belong to the list of ANSM[5] devices.

DEFINITION.–

The European Union defines a medical device as any instrument, apparatus, appliance, software, material or other article, whether used alone or in combination, together with any accessories, including the software intended by its manufacturer to be used specifically for diagnostic and/or therapeutic purposes and necessary for its proper application, intended by the manufacturer to be used by human beings for the purpose of:

– diagnosis, prevention, monitoring, treatment or alleviation of disease;

– diagnosis, monitoring, treatment, alleviation of, or compensation for an injury or disability;

– investigation, replacement or modification of the anatomy or a physiological process;

– control of conception;

– which does not achieve its principal intended action in or on the human body by pharmacological, immunological or metabolic means, but which may be assisted in its function by such means (European directive 93/42/CEE).

---

4 A product labeled "CE" meets certain technical standards and acquires the right to free movement all across the European Union.
5 ANSM: French National Agency for the Safety of Medicine and Health Products (*Agence nationale de sécurité du médicament et des produits de santé*).

Furthermore, everything depends on the manufacturer's intention; if the user demands reimbursement from their health insurance company, they will be evaluated by the responsible authorities, e.g. the National Authority for Health (HAS) in France.

To ensure the standardization of these connected medical devices, the implementation of reference documents and a good practices guide will allow all the actors in connected health, m-health and telemedicine (healthcare professionals, healthcare facilities, manufacturers or users, the public authorities, etc.) to receive help:

– targeting all the critical parameters that must be examined before buying or recommending a connected device to a patient;

– allowing the public authorities to make a decision on whether regulation is necessary.

The Food and Drug Administration (FDA) recently took a step in the direction of greater regulation by looking at the reliability of the measuring methods on mobile medical applications. It requires the developers of medical applications to implement the same risk-management approach used to ensure the safety and efficiency of other medical devices.

1.2.2. Connected objects not having the status of medical devices; they do not necessarily have a medical purpose

This category is made up of all those connected objects that are not medical devices, namely because the manufacturer did not want this.

NOTE.– Let us take the example of a blood pressure monitor. If the device's purpose is solely to provide its user with a numeric value, then this is a connected device and nothing else. Its developer should, nevertheless, start the CE certification or branding process before putting it on the market. However, if this connected object is used to follow a chronic disease and provide diagnosis advice, the unit is a connected medical device.

1.3. The actors in the ecosystem of a connected medical device

It is an entire ecosystem where we find:

– healthcare professionals: the medical auxiliaries made up of healthcare, reeducation and readaptation professions (speech therapist, dietician, etc.) and medical professions (doctor, dentist, etc.). In most cases, they are the recipients of the patient's health data with the aim to become involved in the remote medical care process;

– the governance or responsible authorities in healthcare. In this category we find: medical device (MD) standardization organizations (FDA, CE branding, etc.), the Ministry of Health – the economic and finance minister etc. – administration supervision (ARS, OMEDIT, HAS, ANSM, etc.), the National Health Insurance Fund for Employees (CNAMTS) in France, supervised by the CMS "Center for Medicare and Medicaid Services" in the United States, etc.;

– health establishments that are made up of non-profit healthcare establishments in the private sector (e.g. centers for the fight against cancer), other healthcare establishments in the public sector, long-term care establishments;

– the manufacturers or developers of connected medical devices. Here, we find the providers of complementary functionalities who propose the functionalities of the software, its flexibility, the conditions of use, the technical quality, the ability to provide or store data, etc., to the device's manufacturer.

NOTE.– Let us take the example of a connected non-contact infrared thermometer. The providers of functionality will give the manufacturer the data-visualization system in the form of an individual's daily temperature curves. A manufacturer of the mobile terminal (Samsung, Apple, etc.) will ensure the sale of the products (pharmacies and other companies).

– health data hosts provide physical support (a server) for the storage of health data. They make health data available to the people who are entrusted with them, all while respecting medical confidentiality subject to criminal sanctions;

– the community of users is made up of all patients, family members and their loved ones who use the connected medical device. They can share data with a healthcare professional. They can follow their health parameters to improve care. They can also encourage one another when there are goals to be achieved;

– third parties include all parties who could have access in one way or another to the patient's personal health data; this may be, for instance, scientific researchers furthering their studies on difficult pathologies.

The Digitization of Health

2.1. Definitions of basic concepts

Health applications magnify the quantified self (QS) phenomenon. They constitute the foundation of e-health.

2.1.1. *The quantified self*

The QS movement is "a movement to incorporate technology into data acquisition on aspects of a person's daily life in terms of inputs (food consumed, quality of surrounding air), states (mood, arousal, blood oxygen levels) and performance, whether mental or physical".[1] This movement is founded on the idea that nothing can be improved that cannot be quantified. At the crossroads of telehealth and well-being services, this measurement of oneself involves recording and sharing personal data connected to one's way of life and health. These are practices that illustrate a new relationship with the body and they are likely to further develop our ways of understanding health.

The QS movement was launched in California in 2007 by two editors of *Wired* magazine, Gary Wolf and Kevin Kelly, who hoped to democratize data-monitoring tools. According to Wolf, four large developments allowed for the emergence of this movement: the popularization of smartphones, the advent of social media, the reduction of sensor costs and the onset of cloud computing. In short, QS could never have existed without the advent of open

---

1 Definition from: https://en.wikipedia.org/wiki/Quantified_Self.

data and the softening of the legislation that ensued from it. Companies understood that it was no longer possible to legitimately collect all of this information without proposing a certain restitution to the people concerned.

There are three kinds of QS tools:

– mobile applications: always within easy reach, these allow most personal data (physical activities, health data, etc.) to be recorded;

– sensors: objects worn on one's person (clips, bracelets, watches, etc.) or that are located within the home (scales, a blood pressure monitor, etc.). They can capture, store, analyze and display data;

– Websites: they gather information relevant to our QS process.

2.1.2. *Personal data*

When dealing with personal data (PD), the person responsible for processing the data must conform to their country's pertinent laws, e.g. Law No. 78-17[2] in France. On the one hand, they must ensure that the purpose of the process is defined and that the PD collected are pertinent with regard to this purpose; the data must then be deleted at the end of a determined period. On the other hand, this person must be sure that the people concerned are informed and can exercise their rights (opposition, access, rectification and deletion). It is preferable to assess whether these rights are taken into consideration at the organizational level and whether the exercising of these rights is effective.

2.1.3. *Telemedicine*

In France, telemedicine is defined and supervised according to the HPST[3] law from July 21, 2009. This law defines telemedicine in the French Code of Public Health as:

"A form of remote medical practice using information and communication technologies. It connects, with each other or with a patient, one or more health professionals, which must

---

2 Law no. 78-17 from January 6 1978 concerning computer science, files and freedoms.
3 The "Hospital, Patients, Health, Territories" law (HPST).

include a medical professional and, where appropriate, other professionals providing their care to the patient.

It helps establish a diagnosis, to provide, for a patient at risk, preventative or post-treatment monitoring, to request specialist advice, to prepare a therapeutic decision, to prescribe medication, prescribe or to perform services or acts or to conduct monitoring of the patient's condition. The definition of telemedicine procedures and their conditions for implementing and financial provision are determined by decree, taking into account the deficiencies in the provision of care due to geographic isolation and insularity"[4].

Below are the five medical actions related to telemedicine, performed remotely by means of a device using information and communication technologies:

– teleconsultation: this allows a medical professional to provide a patient with remote consultation. The presence of a health professional can help the patient throughout this consultation;

– tele-expertise: this allows a medical professional to ask for the view of one or more medical experts using elements from the patient's medical records;

– medical telesurveillance: this allows a medical professional to remotely interpret the data necessary for a medical follow-up on a patient in order to make decisions on his or her care;

– this decree also defines the conditions for application, wherein four rules must be respected:

- the person's rights: as with all medical actions, the act of telemedicine requires the patient's prior information and his or her consent to be treated. Once the prior information has been gathered, the exchange of medical data between health professionals who take part in a telemedicine act, regardless of the communication support, no longer requires the receipt of formalized consent except in the case of data storage. In this case, the receipt of consent can be virtual. The patient retains the right of rebuttal at all times;

---

4 Definition taken from: http://www.ceom-ecmo.eu/sites/default/files/documents/simon-lucas_trad_en1.pdf.

- the identification of the actors involved: the health professional must be authenticated and have access to the medical data necessary to treat the patient. The patient must be identified and, when the situation requires it, benefit from the education or preparation necessary for the use of the telemedicine device;

- the telemedicine act must be reported in the medical record: in the medical record, note should be made of the *compte rendu* of the performance, the acts and medical prescriptions effected, the identify of the health professionals, the date and time of the act and, where applicable, mishaps;

- the responsibility of the telemedicine act: the telemedicine act is managed by obligatory medical insurance when it is written on the list of acts undertaken as per article L162-1-7 of the French social security code.

– the conditions of this care are defined in the national conventions concluded between health professionals and the public powers. This includes doctors, dental surgeons, midwives, medical auxiliaries, nurses, masseurs, physiotherapists, medical analysis laboratories and medical transport companies. Private healthcare establishments are also included, as well as health centers. Finally, the text includes medical devices, tissues and cells as soon as they become involved in the framework of a telemedicine act.

2.2. Toward a convergence of the connected objects market

How to think about taking one's medicine? How to live better with one's disease? How to insure oneself for remote care? To respond to these questions, a multitude of health applications are now available to patients. It is interesting to study the evolution of this new market.

2.2.1. *Estimates from the connected objects market*

For the company ABI Research, the global market for mobile connected objects will explode with the general public and see a growth from 16 billion connected objects among us in 2014 to 41 billion in 2020.

Xerfi France estimates that the value of the market for connected objects for health and home will increase by 50% per year between 2013 and 2016.

It was worth 150 million in 2016, namely 3% of the high-tech expenditures in France (vs. 1% in 2013). According to Xerfi's experts, connected watches (in health) and domestic solutions with a box (in the home) will monopolize the first places. The future will go through tight collaboration between manufacturers.

2.2.2. Estimates from the connected health market

This is a market that brings numerous actors together from very different environments such as laboratories, mutual insurance companies, etc. Its rise is the result of several phenomena: aging populations, the need for patient information, obesity, a doctor shortage and the treatment of chronic diseases.

A study conducted by Float Mobile Learning shows that in the United States, "88% of doctors wish some of their patients would monitor their state of health at home". Chad Udell, director of Float Mobile Learning, states "mHealth offers enormous opportunities for people to be more involved in the follow-up of their health and well-being". These intelligent objects represent a major improvement in the conditions for practising medicine and an increase in efficiency.

According to a study conducted by Grand View Research[5] in 2016, "73 million health objects are spread across the world". According to this same study, in 2020 there will be 161 million.

This growth will be inspired by the increase in the average age of the world population, the prevalence in certain countries of patients requiring regular follow-ups and the growing demand for quantifiable solutions for getting back in shape.

In France, Xerfi shows that the "e-health market is worth 2.4 billion euros and is counting on a progression from 4 to 7% per year until 2017". As such, there is talk of the "patient 2.0", an active, connected and informed patient concerning his or her state of health. This patient participates in the search for information, diagnosis, decision making and treatment. Moreover, a

---

5 Source: http://ideas.microsoft.fr/sante-connectee-big-data-iot-5-chiffres-ecteur-mutation/#MoxM fP5JYoJWAv8x.97.

study by TNS Sofres indicates that "one in two French citizens has already used the Internet to search for or share health information and nearly 30% had mobile use". According to this same source, e-health "enthusiasts" are primarily women, more educated and tend to have above-average monthly incomes.

PART 2

Analysis and Cartography of the Risks Linked to Connected Object Usage

3

Project Management

3.1. Research question

Most connected medical devices, such as connected "non-contact" thermometers, allow an input, for example temperature, to be taken by pressing a button at the front of the device and, upon pressing the button again, the "data" to be transferred to a smartphone or tablet via Bluetooth, Wifi, etc. The data is instantly transmitted to the server where it is processed, stored and then sent back to the smartphone to be displayed. No medical data is stored on the smartphone.

The devices' applications (based on iOS or android operating systems) allow the development of the input and its indicators to be followed. Similarly, it is possible to share data with a health professional, one's family or with medical research centers. It is thus a matter of connected medical devices.

Finally, it will also be noted that certain thermometers also allow the ambient temperature or the surface temperature of, for example, bathwater, a bottle or food to be checked.

Putting such devices on the market raises significant concerns relative to the production, storage and exploitation of health data gathered by the user (who may also be the patient). Their aim is to eventually transmit the data to health professionals. After being rendered anonymous and once the user has given their informed consent; the data can also be transmitted to the manufacturers of medical devices or even to epidemiological centers. This gives rise to questions of data integrity, confidentiality and security.

What are the risks that can be linked to the use of a connected medical device?

To respond to this question, we are going to offer you a cartography and comprehensive analysis of the risks linked to the use of connected medical devices.

3.2. Goal of the study

The goal of this study is to perform a comprehensive risk analysis (CRA) [DER 14] in regards to the use of a connected medical device.

NOTE.– CRA is an analytical, inductive and semiquantitative method. Its aim is to identify the scenarios leading to an undesired event when the system displays a danger.

To do this, the primary steps are as follows:

– formalizing the cartography of the dangerous situations after having identified:

  - the dangers and dangerous elements,

  - the dangerous situations and vulnerable elements;

– formalizing the cartography of the scenarios that require:

  - the identification, analysis and evaluation of the risks created by each dangerous situation,

  - the definition and consolidation of the initial and residual risk-reduction actions;

– synthesizing and analyzing the results of the data.

3.3. Scope

The scope of this study is the use of the connected non-contact thermometer by users. The process studied starts from the taking of a person's temperature with the device up until the transmission of the data received in the mobile terminal (smartphone, computer, tablet, etc.) to health professionals.

The characteristics of the users: This is a connected medical device whose users are primarily patients, the public and health professionals.

3.4. Role of the risk manager

The risk manager will allow good practices to be optimized by going through:

– The definition of a robust risk-management policy and the implementation of appropriate devices of analysis and understanding. This policy will aim:

- to identify *a priori* the risks likely to occur during the functioning of our system;

- to create a cartography of the dangerous situations from two generic dangers;

- to establish the different scenarios capable of leading to a feared event (or accident);

- to evaluate the likelihood of these occurring and the gravity of their consequences;

- to evaluate the criticalities;

- to formalize risk cartographies;

- to identify the major risks;

- to define, draft and consolidate a risk-reduction action plan.

– The preventative actions that will allow:

- the identification of the critical paths;

- the proposal of a participatory process;

- the identification of alternative solutions, as well as the application of residual rights and contractual penalties;

- the clarification of the different responsibilities;

- the establishment of scheduled alarms and abnormal performance alarms to alert the operators in the case of controllable or uncontrollable instability in project management.

Comprehensive Risk Analysis Process

4.1. Comprehensive risk analysis system

This stage involves describing and modeling the system and then defining the dangers to which the system is exposed; finally, the dangers/systems interactions are assessed. Description and modeling require that we undertake a functional analysis of our study.

4.1.1. *Functional analysis*

A functional analysis was performed in order to systematically identify the objectives to be attained by the study and thus the processes to be considered. This allows the aims of the study to be defined, to ensure that an existing need is being responded to, and, by precisely delimiting the field of study, the correct need to be defined. Thus, performed at the start of the project, a functional analysis allows the definition of all of the components of the system to be processed and the fundamental need of the system to be identified.

4.1.1.1. *External functional analysis*

We started by expressing the fundamental need of the user of the system studied with the help of an external functional analysis, creating a "bull chart" schematic. This name is linked to its appearance. This method of analysis allows reasoning in relation to the expressed purposes of the system and/or the subproduct, independently of the solutions, in order to study the expected functions and services, to examine the real constraints and to identify the desired performances. It limits the risk of omission or of "going off on a tangent" and it encourages innovations. This is a process that involves responding to the three following questions:

– Whom or what does the system serve?

– Upon whom or what does the system act?

– To what end? To do what?

For this study, our product is the use of connected non-contact thermometers and our system is telemedicine. The bull system "telemedicine" is represented in the following way (see Figure 4.1).

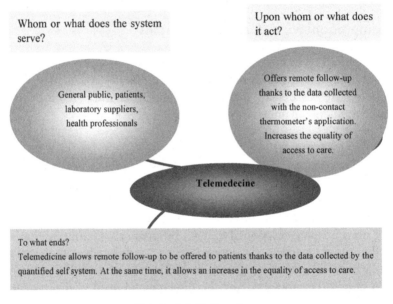

Figure 4.1. *Bull system*

Validity check

Cause: Why does this need exist?

Because the patient needs to be put into remote contact with one or several health professionals through a connected medical device.

Goal: To do what? To what end?

– to establish a diagnosis and ensure patient follow-up;

– to reduce the constraints linked to patients moving;

– to ask a distant and limitedly available specialist for advice;

– to enable caregiving or acts of care.

Stability over time

– *Possibility of disappearance:* There will always be need for remote patient care.

– *Possibility of reinforcement:* The development of new information and communication technologies and particularly the growth of connected medical devices. The stability check on the product over time is validated.

The bull product "connected non-contact thermometer" is represented as follows (see Figure 4.2).

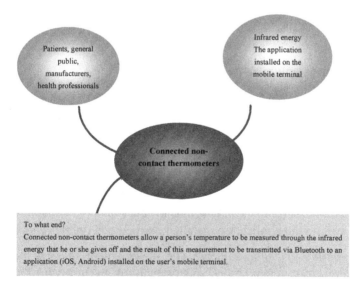

Figure 4.2. *Bull product*

Validity check

In order to validate the expression of our need, the three following questions now remain to be answered:

Cause: Why does this need exist?

Because the user needs to have a simple-to-use device, very user-friendly, easy to handle, with every accessory, and which does not require additional tasks to be performed.

In addition to this simplicity aspect comes that of the speed to implement the device, in the sense that the non-contact thermometer allows the user to see the temperature measurement in less than a second.

Finally, this need exists to allow the user to have a non-invasive medical security device that measures the body temperature without intrusion into the body.

Goal: To do what? To what end?

Connected infrared thermometers allow users to have quantified data about their temperature and to transmit this to their smartphone, which allows them to:

– monitor the evolution of their body temperature;

– monitor their body's performance;

– specify temperature anomalies;

– digitize and collect temperature data;

– obtain an interpretation of the data collected (the quantified self).

Stability over time

 – *Possibility of disappearance:* Users will always have to use connected non-contact thermometers to measure their temperature remotely (non-invasive measurement) and to transmit their data via Bluetooth or Wifi, RFDI, 3G etc., to the application installed on their cell phone or tablet.

 – *Possibility of reinforcement:* The development of new information and communication technologies and particularly the growth of connected medical devices.

NOTE.– Stability checks on the system and the product over time are validated. The need is permanent. Our study, which involves performing a cartography of the risks linked to the use of connected non-contact thermometers, is *a priori* worth being pursued.

4.1.1.2. *Definition of the functions of need*

The table of the definitions of functions allows the different functions revealed by the octopus diagram to be characterized. This allows the translation, through conception demands, of the real need regarding connected non-contact thermometers.

4.1.1.3. *Internal functional analysis*

In order to describe the system of the study, we created a functional tree allowing the system to be divided into different functions. These functions were then segmented into phases and subphases to the level of detail pertinent to the analysis and elaboration of the danger cartography.

The figures below present this system modeling based on the RELIASEP[1] method, which searches for the necessary subfunctions using the need expressed in terms of functions. It is strongly oriented toward functioning safety. It also concentrates on the "entries", "transformations" and "outputs" of each function by considering the performance criteria and the constraints. The RELIASEP method offers segmentation of the principal function or need into three phases, classically:

– capturing the flow;

– transforming the flow;

– transmitting the flow.

In the scope of this study, the principal function of our system "management of risks linked to the functioning of the non-contact thermometer" was segmented into three large subfunctions:

– the "capturing the flow" phase corresponds to "measuring the user's temperature";

– the "transforming the flow" phase corresponds to "visualizing the measurements on the application (on the telephone)";

– the "transmitting the flow" phase corresponds to "sharing measurement data".

---

1 RELIASEP is a method developed by the Société Européenne de Propulsion (SEP). Its goal is to facilitate studies during a system's life cycle by precisely determining the need to be satisfied.

Entities	Identification/ constraining functions (CF)	Name of the function
(Required) security – non-contact thermometers	CF1	Respect the security rules linked to the functioning and use of connected non-contact thermometers. Such as the specific precautions described in the device's user manual
Ergonomics – non-contact thermometers	CF2	Ensure simplicity of use
Autonomy – non-contact thermometers	CF3	Have a duration of use compatible with the duration of the material used
Environmental– non-contact thermometers	CF4	Respect the environment of use
Social responsibility – connected non-contact thermometers	CF5	Ensure data confidentiality
	CF6	Reliability and autonomy
	CF7	Hygienic
Resistance – non-contact thermometers	CF8	Resist minor drops
	CF9	Resist high temperatures
	CF10	Resist elevated humidity
Commercialization – non-contact thermometers	CF11	Cost of acquisition; cost of maintenance; cost of upkeep

Table 4.1. *Constraint functions*

Based on what has previously been done, the modeling of the functional tree from our study goes through the implementation of the constraining and performative functions that we will find in Tables 4.1 and 4.2.

Entities	Identification/ performance functions (P)	Name of the function
Upkeep and storage of non-contact thermometers	P1	Ensure a minimum of education to users for upkeep, use and maintenance of thermometers.
	P2	Offer users a device compatible with certain storage conditions
Environment of use of non-contact thermometers	P3	Provide the right measurement
	P4	Be located at a precise distance from the area where the measurement is to be taken. Certain developers propose taking the temperature at the temporal artery or on the forehead.
	P5	Provide the right profile
	P6	Provide the right IP address
Social responsibility – connected non-contact thermometers	P7	Precision of measurements
	P8	Data integrity
Commercializ ation	P9	Guarantee the device

Table 4.2. *Performance functions*

Using the method mentioned above (RELIASEP), we are going to start the segmentation of the principal function into three phases: capturing the flow, transforming the flow and transmitting the flow.

The "capturing the flow" function corresponds to the "measuring body temperature" phase (see Figure 4.4).

The "transforming the flow" function, on the other hand, corresponds to the "visualizing the measurements (on the application) on the telephone" phase (see Figure 4.5).

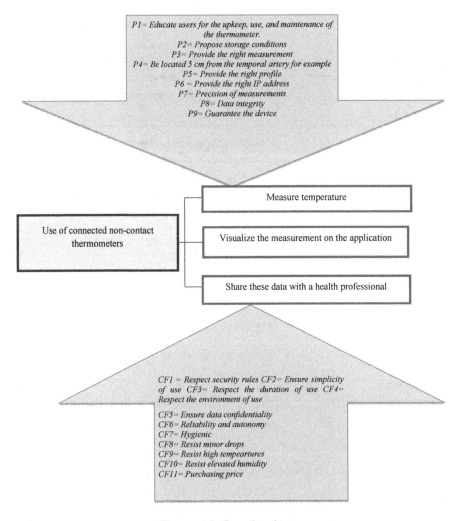

Figure 4.3. *Functional tree*

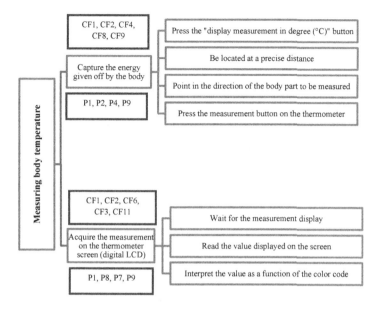

Figure 4.4. *Segmentation of the function, measuring body temperature*

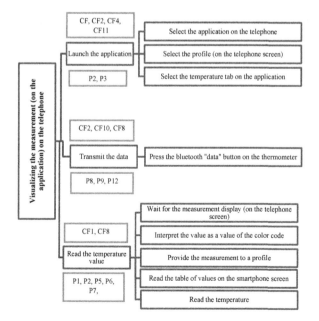

Figure 4.5. *Segmentation of the function, visualizing the measurements (on the application) on the telephone*

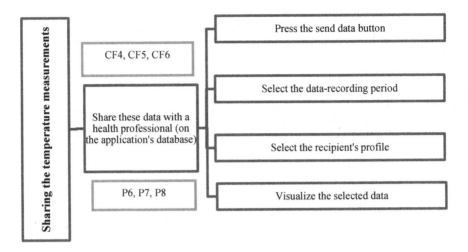

Figure 4.6. *Segmentation of the function, sharing temperature measurements*

Finally, the "transforming the flow" function corresponds to the "sharing the temperature measurements" phase (see Figure 4.6).

Once this step is completed, the comprehensive risk analysis (CRA) system then continues in two stages:

– elaborating the danger cartography: by using a preestablished list of generic dangers to state the specific dangers to which the studied system is exposed, as well as the dangerous elements;

– elaborating the dangerous situation cartography: by locating the interactions between the system elements and the dangerous elements and quantifying these interactions.

4.1.2. *Value and analysis notion approach*

The term value is employed in various domains (health, economics, finance, culture, etc.). However, we can say that first and foremost, what this has in common in every specialty is that it designates the assessment of an object, thereby allowing for judgment.

The AFNOR NF-X-150 norm defines the analysis of value in these terms: "The analysis of value is a method of [corporate] competition, organized and creative, aiming to satisfy the need of the user [client] through a specific design process [of products, systems, services, etc.], simultaneously functional, economic and multidisciplinary. It is an operational method to incite and organize innovation".

The fundamental principle of this method is questioning a product or service. This is the reason why we found it necessary for our study on connected non-contact thermometers to do an analysis allowing us to:

– determine the purposes of the product and/or service;

– shed light on the utility of certain functions;

– determine the cost of the device.

4.1.3. Risk-value balance

In the health domain, the term benefit-risk balance is often used during a diagnostic choice. This allows the proper optimization of medical and pharmaceutical acts. It can be illustrated with the following schema:

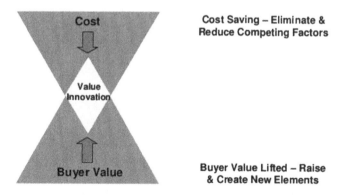

Figure 4.7. *Benefit risks balance*

Using all the assessment data, the benefit-risk balance for a medical procedure is evaluated, first at the collective level. This is generally the one used by the government to decide whether a treatment, device or even a law is authorized.

This notion of risk balance always leads the industrial actors to place the user at the center of all considerations.

4.1.4. *User experience*

Stemming from the human sciences and the ergonomic process, user experience makes it possible to determine the level of satisfaction related to the use of the functions on the one hand and the way of making them develop in terms of shape (functional response), content (function or service in and of itself, its name, description) and the manner of accessing it on the other. The usage criteria can be organized as presented in Table 4.3.

Term	Content
Acceptability	Does this respond to a need in my daily life?
Accessibility	Can I really use this?
Learnability	Can I try it and learn to use it?
Usability	Under what conditions can I use it?
Utility	Of what use is it for me?

Table 4.3. *Constraint functions*

Putting connected objects on the market offers users an original experience that brings man (the user) closer to the machine (connected object) linked to use. The choice of the connected object, its design, the technology used and the service provided have been strategically reconsidered to respond to clients' needs.

For example, connected medical devices allow self-measurement and provide the possibility of adding data, visualizing it and having a comprehensive interpretation of one's health indicators. The user can even set a goal to achieve. We continue our study with the implementation of the dangerous situation cartography.

4.1.5. Danger cartography

The danger cartography was performed using the generic dangerous from a collective task performed by professionals in the GRS[2] master class of 2009–2010 at the Ecole Centrale Paris "generic health danger cartography". For our study, 24 generic dangers and 54 specific dangers have been checked, including:

– image danger: media, public, press;

– insecurity danger: physical, logical, IT;

– client danger: potential users, patient, health professional;

– management danger: organization, resources;

– technological: technological observation, innovation;

– programming danger: update planning;

– financial danger: sales budget, revenue;

– communication danger: internal, external, and patient;

– legal danger: civil and criminal responsibility, patient rights;

– local and infrastructure danger: telemaintenance, electricity;

– material and equipment danger: data-storage unit;

– information system danger: mobile terminal application;

– physicochemical danger: thermal, radiation, biological, mechanic.

---

2 GRS = Specialized Masters in Risk Management and Security of Establishments and Health Networks (*Mastère Spécialisé Gestion des Risques et de la Sécurité des établissements et réseaux de santé*).

Table 4.4 presents the danger cartography from our study.

Generic Dangers	Specific Dangers	Dangerous Events or Elements
Political	National	Unfamiliarity with legislation (standards, laws, decrees, and directives) concerning device usage
	CNIL[3]	Unfamiliarity with the development of regulations
Environmental	Natural	Heatwave (temperature >40°C, humidity <30%), solar flare
		Fire, explosion
	Technological	Distrubance of the equipment's electromagnetic compatibility (EMC)
	Sanitary	Epidemic, pandemic
Insecurity	IT	Unlawful access, identity theft
	Logical	Viral attack
	Physical	Device destruction (or theft)
Image	Public, media, press	Waves of negative opinions concerning the technology proposed by the laboratory
		Spread of a serious, undesirable event connected to the use of the connected medical device
Clients	Users	Refusal to transmit data through the application
	Patients	Anxiety, depression, pressure from stress
		Bodily or visual fatigue
		Difficulty for elderly, chronically ill, and disabled people becoming familiarized with the device
	Health professionals	Invalid creation of the patient record
		Improper management of health data
		Lack of knowledge about good practices in telehealth, telemedicine, e-health, etc.

---

3 *Commission Nationale de l'Informatique et des Libertés* (National Commission on Informatics and Liberty); a French regulatory body to ensure that data privacy law is applied to the collection, storage, and use of personal data.

Management	Organization	Absence of a quality system (for the implementation of protocols, procedures, work instructions, etc.)
		Absence of or improper management of non-conformities
	Resources	Absence of technical competencies to manage post-marketing vigilance problems
Programming	Update planning	Absence of application updates
		Non-functional cellphone (following regular bugs)
Technological	Innovation	Failure to review the device's user guide
	Technological observation	Use of end-of-life technology
		Management does not have access to the information pertaining to the latest technological advances
Communication and crises	Internal communication	Weak or absent oral communication between services, corporatists (marketing, production, logistics)
	Patient communication	Lack of explanation of the device's method of use
Social	Personal	Patient isolation
Ethical and deontological	Confidentiality	Lack of confidentiality
	Human dignity	Lack of respect for intimacy and human dignity
	Transparency	Failure to communicate useful information to patients
Legal	User rights	Failure to receive consent from the patient and health professional
	Regulation	Application installed on the mobile terminal is not declared to the CNIL
		Failure to keep personal data
	Civil and criminal responsibility	Violation of professional secrecy
Financial	Sales budget	Underestimation of the budget allocated to the product
	Revenue	Under- or overestimation of sales projections

	Cost of acquisition	Price of the device too high
Economic	Cost of maintenance	Price of maintenance too high
Commercial	Warranties	Sale of the device without warranty agreement
	Competition	Inaccurate estimates of competitors' prices
Infrastructure and local	Electricity	Blackout
	Telemaintenance	Maintenance not handled by laboratory personnel
Materials and equipment	Data-storage unit	Exceeding function limits
		Unprotected storage components
		Impossible data restoration
	(Virtual) servers	Unavailability of servers
		Server's inability to read or handle errors
		Hacking of server by malicious actor
		Lack of specific back-ups related to virtual operations
Information system	Application (on the smartphone)	Information leak
		Malicious program on the telephone
		Partial or total deletion of the application
		Spread of a virus
	Computer network (Bluetooth)	Connecting to an unsecure Bluetooth network
		Concealed data transfer
		Disconnection from network
		Network failure
	(Data) hosting	Stolen data
Project and studies	Product (or connected medical device)	Insufficiently specified and/or absent performance control indicators
		Concept incompatible with client needs
		Flaw concerning ergonomics and device size
	Planification	Review of defective material
	Delivery	Improper or absent delivery management
		Unavailability of devices on the market

Operational	Quality control	Device-quality problems identified after release onto the market
		Device production tool does not meet quality standards
	Activities	Failure to respect production specifications
		Informal exploitation of performance indicators
	Maintenance	Lack of device maintenance
	After-sales service	Failure to provide a timely response to client demands
		Forgetting to respond to client demands
		The devices' storage locations are ill-defined
Human factor	Individual (user)	Lack of respect for device maintenance rules
		Transmission of data to the incorrect recipient
		User misuse
		Lack of respect for device instructions
		No mastery of the recharging process for the connected non-contact thermometer
		Abnormal use of the application or device
	Identity monitoring	Error with the application's access codes
		Error attributing data to a profile (unrelated profile)
Professional	Biological	Presence of an energy source
Physicochemical	Electrical	Sub-voltage device
		Corrosion
	Thermic	Extreme heat
		Extreme cold
	Biological	Unfamiliarity with the different types of radiation from the human skin
		Damaged or dead skin
	Radiation	Device ionization
		Electrocution (after using a defective USB cable)
	Mechanical	Significant acoustic vibrations
		Device falling from base or violent shock

Products	Functional failures	Delayed function
		Accelerated function
		Untimely functioning
		Intermittent functioning
		Loss of one or several device functions
		Lack of supervision of the device's system functions
		Drift in the functional parameters (abnormal quantity of energy captured by the optical probe)

Table 4.4. *Danger cartography. For a color version of this table, see www.iste.co.uk/beyala/health.zip*

4.1.6. *Cartography of dangerous situations*

The cartography of dangerous situations is performed by cross-referencing the system phases and the list of dangers. This superposition allows the interaction between dangers and the vulnerability of the system's elements to be assessed. This interaction is expressed according to a three-level scale.

Three levels of vulnerability are distinguished. These are presented in Table 4.5.

In the case of our study, we have:

– 76 dangerous situations with priority index 1;

– 93 dangerous situations with priority index 2;

– 62 dangerous situations with priority index 3.

Priority index	Dangers/System Interaction	Analysis, evaluation, and treatment decision
0	No interaction	
1	Strong to very strong	Immediately
10	Strong to very strong	Later
2	Weak to medium	Subsequently

Table 4.5. *Scale of dangers/system interaction. For a color version of this table, see www.iste.co.uk/beyala/health.zip*

Table 4.6 presents the cartography of dangerous situations from our study project.

Cartography and management of risks linked to the use of a connected non-contact thermometer

76   93   60

Generic dangers	Specific dangers	Dangerous events or elements	(A) Activating Body mode	(A) Positioning at a precise distance	(A) Pointing in the direction of the temporal artery	(A) Pressing the button on the thermometer	(A) Waiting for the measurement display	(A) Reading the value displayed on the screen	(A) Interpreting the value by means of the color code	(B) Selecting the application on the telephone	(B) Selecting the profile on the telephone screen	(B) Selecting the temperature tab	(B) Pressing the Bluetooth "data" button on the application	(B) Waiting for the measurement to be displayed on the telephone screen	(B) Interpreting the value by means of the color code	(B) Attributing the temperature to a profile	(B) Reading the table of measurements on the telephone screen	(B) Viewing the temperature curve displayed	(C) Pressing the send data button	(C) Selecting the saving period of the data	(C) Viewing the selected data	(C) Selecting the sending period of temperature data	(C) Selecting the recipient
Political	National	Unfamiliarity with legislation				2				2			2								1		1
	CNIL	Unfamiliarity with developments in regulations											10								1		1
Environmental	Natural	Heat wave Solar flare				1							10										
		Fire, explosion				1																	
	Technological	Disturbance of the field		1	10	1																	
	Sanitary	Epidemic, pandemic				1																	
Insecurity	IT	Unlawful access, identity theft																			1		1
	Logical	Viral attack									10	2				10	10				1		1
	Physical	Device destruction (or theft)				1				2			2			1						1	

Category	Subcategory	Risk / description	Values
Image	Public, media, press	Negative opinions of the technology	1
		Serious, undesirable event connected to use	1
Clients	Users	Refusal to transmit the data through the application	10, 1, 10, 2, 10
		Anxiety, depression, pressure from stress	10
	Patients	Bodily or visual fatigue	10
		Difficulty familiarizing oneself with the device	1, 1, 10, 2, 1
		Invalid creation of the patient record	10, 2
	Health professionals	Improper management and/or use of health data	2
		Lack of knowledge about good practices in the domain: telehealth, telemedicine, etc.	
		Absence of a quality system	1
Management	Organization	Absence or improper management of nonconformities	1, 10
	Resources	Absence of technical competencies to manage materials vigilance problems	2, 10, 10
		Absence of application updates	1
Programming	Planning updates		1
		Nonfunctional cellphone (following regular bugs)	1

Technological	Innovation	Failure to review the device's user guide	10		10
	Technological observation	Use of end-of-life technology			
		Management does not have access to the information pertaining to the latest technological advances	2		
Communication and crises	Internal communication	Weak or absent oral communication between services	10		
	Patient communication	Lack of explanation			10
Social	Personal	Patient isolation			2
	Transparency	Failure to communicate useful information to patients			1

Table 4.6. *Cartography of dangerous situations. For a color version of this table, see www.iste.co.uk/beyala/health.zip*

4.2. CRA scenario

4.2.1. *Scale of gravity*

The scale of gravity of the consequences (Table 4.7) allows the impact of the dangerous situations on remote care, the physical integrity of the data, the physical integrity of the device and data confidentiality to be defined in terms of harm or damage.

We wish to remind the reader that this scale is made up of the five following levels:

– the G1 class of gravity, which characterizes the absence of an impact on the system's performance or security;

– the G2 and G3 classes of gravity characterize harm concerning the system's performance without an impact on security;

– the G4 and G5 classes of gravity characterize the reduction or failure of the system's security.

The scale was created by the work group by transposing the consequences that may concern each level of gravity for each of the system's factors (users of non-contact thermometers, patient, health professionals). Table 4.7 presents the scale of gravity relative to the present study.

4.2.2. *Scale of likelihood*

This scale allows for the assessment of the occurrence of consequences connected to the realization of a described scenario. It is a tool that allows for the assessment of the probability that the consequences of a feared event may occur. It is made up of five levels of probability defined subjectively by the work group. To create our work scale, estimates were made concerning the frequency with which a user (patient, client, etc.) takes his or her temperature remotely with the thermometer. The scale of likelihood is presented in Table 4.8.

Class of gravity	Title of the class	Index	Title of the consequences
G1	Minor	1	No impact on the activity's performance and security
			11 Unavailability of the device <5 min with no alteration of measurement data
			12 Recovery or correction of the data with no operational difficulty or financial losses
			13 Warning without notice followed by a free proposition for regulation
			14 Client dissatisfaction without demands
G2	Significant (reduced mission)	2	Reduction in the system's performance with no impact on security
			21 Unavailability of the device >5 min with service delay but data recovery
			22 Recovery or correction of data with minor financial losses <500€
			23 Order to stop processing contentious data
			24 Financial losses <500€
G3	Serious (failed mission)	3	Great reduction or failure of the system's performance with no impact on security
			31 Unavailability of the device <10 min + substantial alteration of data
			32 Recovery or correction of data with major financial losses <1,000€
			33 Withdrawal of authorization or lockdown (by the CNIL) of data + amends <3,000€
			34 Financial losses between 500€ and 5,000€

			Reduction of the system's security or integrity
G4	Critical (reduced security)	4	41 Unavailability of the device >10 min with partial data loss
			42 Recovery or correction of data with significant financial losses <2,000€
			43 Complaint followed by a sentence and moderate damages < 100,000€
			44 Financial losses + harm and interests between 5,000€ and 100,000€
			Great reduction or failure of security or loss of the system
G5	Catastrophic (failed security)	5	51 Total unavailability of the device, service failure
			52 Recovery or correction of data with financial losses above 3,000€
			53 Sentence on the manufacturer with financial penalties between 100,000€ and 300,000€
			54 Impossibility of remote care

Table 4.7. *Scale of gravity*

Class of likelihood	Title of the class	V index	Title of the likelihoods	T = The number of times the temperature was taken
L1	Very improbable	1	Less than once by T1	
			T1–>	125 (2 years)
L2	Improbable	2	Between once by T1 and once by T2	
			T2–>	60 (1 year)
L3	Rather probable	3	Between once by T2 and once by T3	
			T3–>	25 (4 months)
L4	Probable	4	Between once by T3 and once by T4	
			T4–>	10 (1 month)
L5	Very probable to certain	5	More than once by T4	

Table 4.8. *Scale of likelihood*

4.2.3. *Criticality matrix*

This is a decision tool relative to the degree of risk acceptability. It characterizes the objective and subjective importance given to the combination (gravity, likelihood). It is made up of three classes of criticality, whose level will determine the nature of the decision to be made concerning the residual risk management. The risk's criticality is defined according to Table 4.9.

The appreciation of the acceptability or unacceptability of the risk is a function of each individual's own aversion to the risk. The criticality matrix (Figure 4.8) constitutes a decision tool and represents the frame of reference for the risk acceptability proper to our study.

Class of criticality	Title of the class	Index	Titles of the decisions and actions
C1	Acceptable as is	1	No action should be taken
C2	Tolerable under supervision	2	A follow-up must be organized in terms of risk management
C3	Unacceptable	3	The situation must be refused. Risk-reduction measures must necessarily be implemented; otherwise, all or part of the activity must be refused.

Table 4.9. *Scale of criticality. For a color version of this table, see www.iste.co.uk/beyala/health.zip*

Figure 4.8. *Frame of reference for risk acceptability. For a color version of this figure, see www.iste.co.uk/beyala/health.zip*

Upon reflection, criticality C3 has been assigned to events:

– whose consequences are serious (G3) and whose likelihood is very probable to certain (L5);

– whose consequences are catastrophic (G5) but whose likelihood is rather improbable (L3), between once per year and once every 4 months.

Furthermore, criticality C2 (tolerable under supervision) and not C3 (unacceptable) has been assigned to events:

– whose likelihood is very probable to certain (L5) even for significant consequences (G2);

– whose consequences are catastrophic (G5) with a very high likelihood (L2);

– whose consequences are critical (G4) with a very high likelihood (L2).

Finally, criticality C1 (acceptable as is) and not C2 (tolerable under supervision) has been assigned to events:

– whose consequences are minor (G1) and whose likelihood is very probable to certain (L5);

– whose likelihood is very improbable (L1) but with catastrophic consequences (G5), particularly "impossibility of remote care".

This is justified by the fact that, in the current cultural and societal context, in the case of the impossibility of remote care via connected non-contact thermometer, the patient can always turn to traditional care. This situation can then be acceptable. It is not conceivable to consider a catastrophic event (very unlikely) for which there is an alternative solution as being unacceptable or tolerable under supervision.

4.2.4. Scale of loss

The notion of loss is translated by the cost of the risk without resolution, that is the amount of harm in the absence of risk management.

Class of loss	Levels	Index	Titles of losses by consequence
P0	None	0	Nothing is done
P1	Slight	1	Very slight loss
P2	Moderate	2	Moderate loss
P3	Significant	3	Significant to very significant loss

Table 4.10. *Description of the classes of loss*

Table 4.11 explains the method to calculate the index for each class of loss from the system studied.

System	Sim[20]	Index of effort		
	%	1	2	3
Measuring the temperature	5%	500	3000	10000
Visualizing the measurements on the application	10%	1500	3000	30000
Sharing these measurement data with a health professional	15%	2500	3000	40000

Table 4.11. *Method to calculate the indices for each class of loss*

4.2.5. Scale of effort

The notion of effort is translated by the cost corresponding to the investment in the risk resolution, that is in the number of risk management actions (human means, technical investments, etc.) to be implemented.

Class of effort	Levels	Index	Titles of efforts by action
E0	None	0	Nothing is done
E1	Slight	1	Very slight to slight effort
			Temporary supervision or action
E2	Moderate	2	Moderate effort
			Periodic supervision or action
E3	Significant	3	Significant to very significant effort
			Continuous supervision or action
			Highest level effort

Table 4.12. *Description of the classes of effort*

To define our scale of effort, several aspects were taken into consideration:

– human costs (salaries in the case of a position that must be replaced, use of internal resources, time working in partnership, etc.);

– external costs (involvement of an external service provider, educational costs, etc.).

System	Sim[20]	Index of losses		
	%	1	2	3
Measuring the temperature	8%	500	1000	10000
Visualizing the measurements on the application	11%	500	1000	30000
Sharing these measurement data with a health professional	15%	500	1000	40000

Table 4.13. *Method to calculate the indices for each class of effort*

Results of the Scenario and Dangerous Situation Analysis

5.1. Dangerous situation analysis

The comprehensive risk analysis of this study allowed us to establish the dangerous situation cartography on all interactions with a priority level of 1 (to be treated immediately). These were the subject of treatment followed by an identification of the accident scenarios. The comprehensive risk analysis allowed us to treat 76 dangerous situations which have been converted into 151 accident scenarios.

5.1.1. *By function*

The following subfunctions: "measuring the temperature" and "sharing these measurement data with a health professional" constitute most of the dangerous situations, 42% and 30%, respectively. The subfunction "visualizing the measurements on the application" only constitutes 27%.

Number of Dangerous Scenarios identified and scenarios analyzed by System element

System		NSD	NSc
1	Measuring the temperature	A	32	64
2	Visualizing the measurements on the application (on the telephone)(B)	B	21	41
3	Sharing these measurement data with a health professional (C)	C	23	46
			76	151

Figure 5.1. *Number of dangerous situations (NDS) and scenarios (NSc) by phase. For a color version of this figure, see www.iste.co.uk/beyala/health.zip*

5.1.2. *By danger*

The dangerous situations are distributed according to dangers in the following way:

– 11% for the danger "information system" (7% of the scenarios);

– 7% for the danger "material and equipment" (8% of the scenarios);

– 8% for the danger "human factor" (9% of the scenarios);

– 9% for the danger "physicochemical" (7% of the scenarios);

– 7% for the danger "clients" (11% of the scenarios).

Number of Dangerous Situations identified and scenarios analyzed by danger

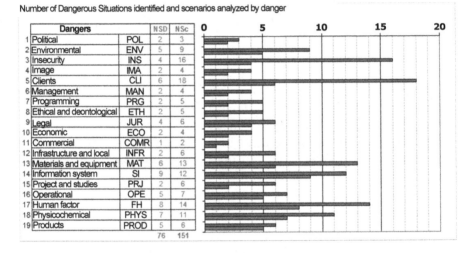

	Dangers		NSD	NSc
1	Political	POL	2	3
2	Environmental	ENV	5	9
3	Insecurity	INS	4	16
4	Image	IMA	2	4
5	Clients	CLI	6	18
6	Management	MAN	2	4
7	Programming	PRG	2	5
8	Ethical and deontological	ETH	2	5
9	Legal	JUR	4	6
10	Economic	ECO	2	4
11	Commercial	COMR	1	2
12	Infrastructure and local	INFR	2	6
13	Materials and equipment	MAT	6	13
14	Information system	SI	9	12
15	Project and studies	PRJ	2	6
16	Operational	OPE	5	7
17	Human factor	FH	8	14
18	Physicochemical	PHYS	7	11
19	Products	PROD	5	6
			76	151

Figure 5.2. *Number of dangerous situations (NDS) and scenarios (NSc) by danger. For a color version of this figure, see www.iste.co.uk/beyala/health.zip*

5.2. Scenario analysis

5.2.1. *Measurements already implemented by certain manufacturers*

Before conducting this study, the manufacturers who ensure the promotion of these connected medical devices had already implemented certain actions aiming to reduce the occurrence of feared events as well as the gravity of their consequences, notably:

– For feared events linked to the information system danger:

- server analysis and reintegration of the data if necessary;

- storage on virtual servers with multiple safeguards on multiple sites;

- regular safeguards on multiple back-ups;

- firewall protocol that allows access to the server ports to be blocked;

- level 7 firewall protocol that allows the presence of viruses to be detected in the software layer.

In the case of memory saturation, the existence of a protocol that uses algorithms to search for orphan data.

– For feared events linked to legal danger:

Implementation of the Fast Healthcare Interoperability Resources (FHIR) data format. This is a data format adapted for the medical domain. Medical data sent are separated from the patient's identity. Within the database (BDD), there is no direct link between patients and their data.

Procurement of the CE Medical classes IIa marking and FDA for the object and application.

5.2.2. Scenario estimation by initial criticity

In the 151 mentioned scenarios concerning the 76 dangerous situations with a priority level of 1, it can be noted here that before treatment, 3% of the scenarios present an unacceptable risk as is, therefore a C3 criticity.

Among these unacceptable initial risks, two take place three times per year. Moreover, three of them take place once per year. Measures were proposed in the risk-reduction action plan.

– 19% have a C2 criticity, therefore tolerable under supervision;

– 78% have a C1 criticity, therefore acceptable as is.

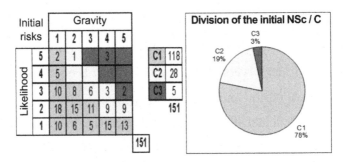

Figure 5.3. *Division of the scenarios (NSc) by the average risks (AR) and by criticity before risk-reduction actions. For a color version of this figure, see www.iste.co.uk/beyala/health.zip*

5.2.3. *Scenario estimation by residual criticity*

After treatment, that is, the implementation of the risk-reduction actions, 3% of the scenarios present a risk that is tolerable under supervision requiring the application of surveillance actions.

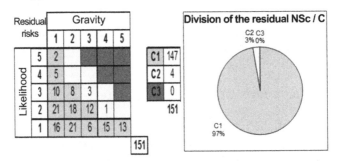

Figure 5.4. *Division of the scenarios (NSc) by the average risks (AR) and by criticity after risk-reduction actions. For a color version of this figure, see www.iste.co.uk/beyala/health.zip*

All of the unacceptable initial risks were reduced because of the measures implemented. We also note that 97% of the scenarios present acceptable risks.

6

Comprehensive Risk Analysis by Subfunction and by Danger

6.1. By subfunction

Comprehensive risk analysis is an ISO 31000 standard method. In the framework of our study, it allows us to take an inventory and analyze the risks from our system's three subfunctions.

6.1.1. Decision diagram

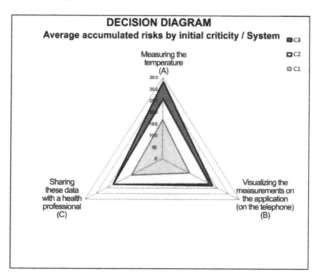

Figure 6.1. *Decision diagram. For a color version of this figure, see www.iste.co.uk/beyala/health.zip*

The decision diagram (Figure 6.1) presents the average accumulated risks for each subfunction by initial criticity. It shows us that phase A, "measuring the temperature", is the most sensitive. It accumulates more risks with a C3 criticity. Then comes phase B, "visualizing the measurements on the application", which accumulates slightly fewer C3 risks than the preceding category. Phase C, "sharing these data with a health professional", is the one that accumulates the least risks.

Phase A, "measuring the temperature", is the most sensitive because it calls on human errors linked to improper handling. The sensor integrated into the thermometer is a microprocessor that generates data on the body, surface or ambient temperature. However, it is not capable of verifying the correlation between past and present data. It is thus the job of users to ensure that they have respected the instructions to avoid the worst-case scenario.

6.1.2. Kiviat diagram

The Kiviat diagram allows minimum, average and maximum risk values to be visualized for each phase of the system studied. Its axes are standardized into average risk indices ranging from 0 to 25. The green dotted line symbolizes the lower limit between the minimum risk and the average risk. It corresponds to the gravity product by likelihood by referring to the criticity matrix. It is equal to 3 (G3xL1).

The red dotted line represents the upper limit between the average risk and the maximum risk, which corresponds to 8 (G3xL3).

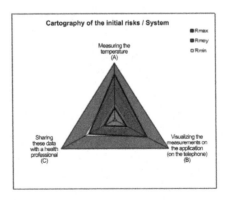

Figure 6.2. KIVIAT diagram of the average initial risks by phase. For a color version of this figure, see www.iste.co.uk/beyala/health.zip

In this study, the maximum risk is 15 (G5xL3). A risk is therefore considered major once the value of its product is greater than or equal to 15. Between 3 and 8, we have a level 1 criticity and above 8 and below 15, a level 2 criticity. As Figure 6.2 shows, all the phases are impacted by the maximum C3 criticity risk. Similarly, the minimum risk spreads across all three phases.

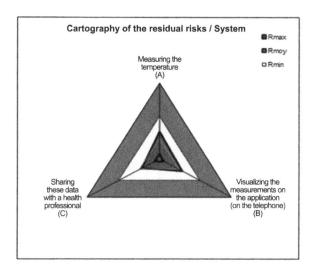

Figure 6.3. *KIVIAT diagram of the average initial and residual risks by phase. For a color version of this figure, see www.iste.co.uk/beyala/health.zip*

After treatment, the maximum risk has a C2 criticity across all three phases. The "measuring the temperature" phase remains a C2 criticity, as does the "visualizing the measurements on the application" phase.

6.1.3. *Farmer diagram*

The farm diagrams (Figure 6.4) allow the average gravities and likelihoods to be visualized for each phase of the system studied. The average gravity of the initial or residual risks corresponds to the sum of the initial or residual gravities divided by the number of scenarios per phase.

The average likelihood of the initial or residual risks corresponds to the sum of the initial or residual likelihoods divided by the number of scenarios per phase. The criticity matrix serves as the foundation for the location of the red and green lines. This diagram has three zones:

– the unacceptable average initial or residual risks are above the red line;

– the average initial or residual risks that are tolerable under supervision are located between the green line and the red line;

– the acceptable average initial or residual risks are located below the green line.

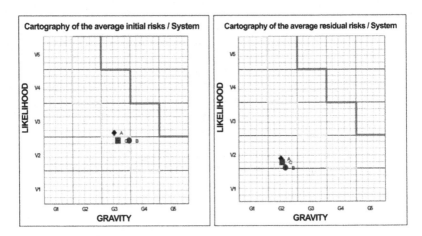

Figure 6.4. *Cartographies of average initial and residual risks by phase. For a color version of this figure, see www.iste.co.uk/beyala/health.zip*

For the system studied, two points stand out:

– the average initial risks for phase A "measuring the temperature" and phase B "visualizing the measurement data on the application" are located in the zone "tolerable under supervision";

– the risk-reduction actions necessary for treatment are a mixture of prevention actions (reduction of the likelihood index) and protection actions (reduction of the gravity index).

6.2. By danger

6.2.1. Decision diagram

Concerning the risks accumulated by initial criticity with regard to our decision diagram of dangers (Figure 6.5), the decision diagram shows a prioritization of the actions on the danger "Clients" and then the danger "Physicochemica" and "Information system", and finally, the danger "Image".

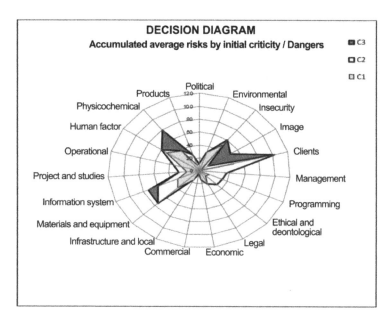

Figure 6.5. *Decision diagram by danger. For a color version of this figure, see www.iste.co.uk/beyala/health.zip*

Vulnerabilities appear at the level of the danger "client" because connected non-contact thermometers constitute a new technology, yet the adoption of such a medical device is influenced by factors that require a strong understanding of the risks. Among these are:

– observability, which allows familarization with a device and therefore the reduction of uncertainty;

– testability, which involves being able to easily try out the thermometer;

– comprehension concerning the device's use or instructions and the utility perceived by the individual, including subjective judgments (social networks, media, etc.).

Furthermore, the physicochemical danger required prioritization of the risk-reduction actions. The world is unqestionably faced with a new product.

There can thus be obstacles during the manufacturing process that will have an impact on the reliability of the device. Passing from a series of tests (like the integration of a so-called "new" probe into the device and the analysis and evaluation of the electromagnetic flow to the surface of the skin in order to improve the precision of the algorithm) to a large series when the product is released into the market and reviewing production procedures and/or protocols are some of the variables that manufacturers of this kind of medical device must manage to overcome the physicochemical risk.

Additionally, the image risk, i.e. everything that can jeopardize the development of the manufacturer's activity, presents a considerable number of vulnerabilities. This shows that the developers should permanently improve measurements that can allow them to better determine the client's expectations and respect the quality of conformity of their proposed technical solutions.

6.2.2. *Kiviat diagram*

The representation of the initial risks by danger through this Kiviat diagram shows that the dangers information system, physicochemical and image have a level 3 criticity with a maximum risk equal to 15.

The risks with a C3 criticity present in the information system danger refer to all sorts of malicious acts.

In fact, once the temperature data of this technology's users go toward a server installed by the manufacturer, one of the principal risks is the use of personal data for fraudulent purposes by malicious actors. It can also be a matter of use aiming to disturb the user's peace of mind through a divulgence of their health data to the general public. Furthermore, the risk of leaking information or pirating of the personal data storage system by cybercriminals is all the more elevated given that these connected non-contact thermometers as connected objects do not necessarily possess software to detect malicious acts.

As for the physicochemical danger, it calls on all the risks linked to the reliability of the sensor. All of these risks have a negative impact on the brand image of the laboratory and the technology it offers.

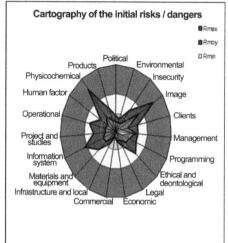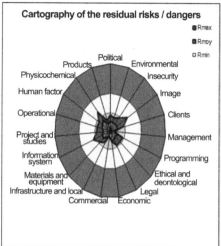

Figure 6.6. *Cartographies of initial and residual risks by danger. For a color version of this figure, see www.iste.co.uk/beyala/health.zip*

Insecurity, material and equipment, clients, management, project and studies, operational, legal, ethical and deontological, have a C2 criticity.

The presence of risks with a C2 criticity particularly resorts to:

– The violation of personal data confidentiality

Respect for people's private lives is a fundamental factor considered by numerous users. Certain manufacturers offer users free secure hosting in a personal health data host. However, the personalization of the application's confidentiality settings, nevertheless, remains a question. Following this example, the CNIL is currently reflecting on the definition of a certification to encourage the creators of e-health applications to better inform users about the use of their personal data. This could even allow them to reassure the clientele and prove their engagement in a relationship of trust.

– Data integrity

This is the determining criterion, as it is the idea of honesty that the consumer attributes to the brand. Commercial, environmental, political and economic have a C1 criticity.

After treatment, the risk-reduction actions bring all the maximum risks to a C2 criticity.

The presence of C1 criticity risks on the political danger is linked to the issue of the absence of a homogeneous standard relative to the treatment of the data collected through a connected medical device "for users who are located outside the European Union".

In fact, within the European Union, directive 95/46/CE[1] is designed to be applied. However, for users located in a country outside the European Union, this standard does not apply. There is currently no commonly accepted definition with the European Union at an "appropriate" security level concerning the processing of health data that could be applied in the case of processing and collecting cross-border data. Thus, for example, a patient located in a member state may be obliged by national rules concerning the protection of data to adopt particular security measures relative to the collection of data through a connected medical device, while this could potentially not be the case in other member states. It is necessary to implement an extra-territorial law on this subject (the transfer and/or processing of data via connected objects having the status of a connected medical device).

A report written by *legal experts from the University of Amsterdam* maintains that the *"Patriot Act*[2]*"* bypasses European laws concerning personal data.

In certain cases, it will force American companies to go against European laws. It is essentially this problem that must be resolved in order to ensure that data storage in Europe remains outside the scope of U.S. requests. This text gives full power to the United States concerning research: all American companies must provide sensitive data demanded by the Federal Administration, no matter where they are stored. Concretely, data hosted on French soil by an American actor can be requested by the National Security Agency (NSA[3]) or another information service without advance notification to the country's authorities or the company in question. This law concerns

---

1 Law relative to the processing and collection of health data like temperature data.
2 The Patriot Act is a law to unite and reinforce the United States by providing the tools necessary to detect and counter terrorism. It does not recognize territoriality.
3 The National Security Agency is a government organization of the U.S. Department of Defense.

and impacts almost all hosting service, safeguard and data storage providers. On the other hand, personal data protection laws do not protect European citizens against extraterritorial laws like those of the United States.

6.2.3. Farmer diagram

The Farmer diagrams (Figure 6.7) allow the average gravities and average likelihoods to be visualized for each family of dangers.

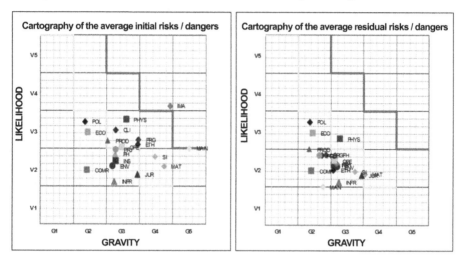

Figure 6.7. *Cartographies of the average initial and residual risks by danger. For a color version of this figure, see www.iste.co.uk/beyala/health.zip*

In the system studied, the danger "Material" is located in the unacceptable zone. This is justified by the fact that following the implementation of risk-reduction actions, all the dangers are located between the acceptable zone and the tolerable under supervision zone.

7

The Scales of Loss and Effort

7.1. Analysis of the scales loss and effort

The diagrams of the costs efforts/risks, shown in Figure 7.1, make a situation visible to us in which the cost of risk treatment is superior to the cost of the losses without treatment. The implementation of the action plan would thus allow political treatment of the risk on the whole system.

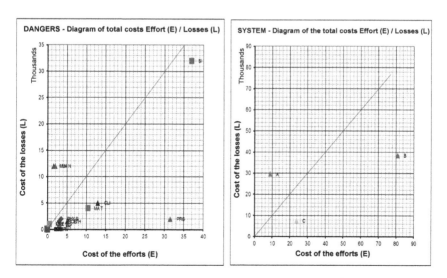

Figure 7.1. *Diagrams of the total costs effort by losses of dangers and phases*

NOTE.– The establishment of a new market such as "connected non-contact thermometry" results in political risk treatment and therefore a strategic stake for manufacturers.

In the scope of technological innovation like that of connected non-contact thermometry, it is normal for the understanding of the risks to become a strategic stake for manufacturers offering this kind of solution. This is a new market that must be given value in a short time (at the risk of being overtaken by one's competitors), with sufficient quality (at the risk of seeing the client turn away), and at an acceptable cost (so that developers earn profit from their products).

In other words, the market for connected medical devices arises from the societal, political, legal, ethical and deontological stakes. The fact that there is governance that considers these aspects beforehand allows for the individual limitation of the negative consequences of a serious undesired event or the impact of a degraded situation, on the one hand, and knowledge of how to act in the face of a risk likely to affect it through its value chain, on the other: particularly its clients, providers, or even transporters, etc. By strategically organizing its observation through the collection of information (e.g. clients' opinions and expectations concerning the product), through its analysis, and through its impact far in advance, starting with research and development (R&D), the company can optimize the value chain of its product.

7.2. List of major risks

Major risks are defined in relation to:

– risks with a C3 criticity;

– average risk index (G × V= 15, 16 and 20);

– catastrophic gravity (G = 5).

According to the results obtained from our risk cartography, the problems that can appear with the use of a connected medical device such as a connected non-contact thermometer display various and diverse natures. They do not all present the same degree of gravity or occurrence. These problems range from instructions that are not applied, not understood, or complex, to incomplete information or an absent, though displayed, functionality, all the way to a calculation or diagnostic orientation error. These concern:

– product dysfunction most often connected to the improper use of the thermometer. This reliability problem most often produces a lack of confidence and credibility for both the brand and the manufacturer;

– greater vulnerability connected to the security of the information system of the device and/or the application appears during the transfer of data to a professional or a third party (remember that all of the user's health data are hosted by the Ministry of Health in a HADS).

– these major risks are summarized in Table 7.1.

7.3. Risk-reduction action plan and catalogue of security parameters

Based on the comprehensive risk analysis scenario, risk-reduction actions have been defined with the expertise of the scientific director. Table 7.2 includes all the files from these risk-reduction actions. These actions cover one or several phases of the system.

The titles of the action files drafted concern the actions to be implemented to reduce the major risks classified as unacceptable from C3 to C2. Their implementation will also allow certain risks not classified as major, with a C2 criticity and therefore tolerable under supervision, to be reduced.

Table 7.3 shows the security parameter files. These files detail the residual risk management actions to be implemented when the residual criticity remains C2. All of these security parameter files constitute the catalogue of security parameters.

For our study, we have three security parameter files listed in Table 7.3.

MR	Dangerous situation	Feared event	Trigger cause	Danger	Subphase
20	Swathes of negative opinions regarding the technology	Drop in sales and sales revenue	Establishment of several points of sale for the device	Image	Measuring the temperature (A)
20	Unfamiliarity with the different types of skin radiation	Unreliable data	Device usage	Physicochemical	Measuring the temperature (A)
15	Spread of a virus through a malicious file	Total loss or modification of sensitive data	Need to use the mobile terminal's application to transfer health data to a professional for remote care	Information system	Visualizing the measurements on the application (on the telephone) (B)
15	Spread of a virus through a malicious file	Third-party complaints	Free access to health data (by unauthorized persons)	Information system	Visualizing the measurements on the application (on the telephone) (B)

Table 7.1. *List of the major risk*

Reference	Risk-reduction action files
A1	Drafting a protocol that allows data to be encrypted by the telephone and decrypted by the server, which alone has the key.
A2	Educating personnel on the external SAV 1 to work together with the development team.
A3	Educating personnel on the quality control (standardization) of products at the warehouse.
A4	Making information campaign forms available to users by e-mail to notify them about critical updates.
A5	Drafting a protocol that allows the simulation of malicious attacks and the identification of vulnerabilities present in the software.
A6	Drafting an automated database cleaning procedure.
A7	Making new quick steps available to users, taking into consideration the aspect of application use on the telephone, tablet or computer.
A8	Drafting a procedure to improve sales forecast management.
A9	Improving the precision of infrared waves by integrating a new probe into the device.
A10	Implementing a system to analyze surface blood flow by camera/probe.
A11	Implementing a protocol to analyze skin composition by camera.
A12	Evaluating the electromagnetic flow on the surface of the skin in order to improve the precision of the algorithm.
A13	Promoting telehealth education for pharmacists or health professionals.
A14	Implementing a strong identification protocol to protect access to the database (for health professionals).
A15	Implementing necessary development of the computer tool to improve storage management.
A16	Drafting a certificate procedure for exchanges with the POPs[1].
A17	Implementing a product launch procedure with all the elements necessary for the launch.

Table 7.2. *The different risk-reduction action files*

1 Post Office Protocols: a type of computer networking and Internet standard *protocol* that extracts and retrieves e-mail from a remote *mail server for access by the host machine* (Definition from *https://www.techopedia.com/definition/5383/post-office-protocol-pop*).

Reference	Security parameter file
P1	Verifying the application of the procedures during production
P2	Verifying the application of the protocol
P3	Monthly audit on the vulnerabilities of the application's information system

Table 7.3. *The different security parameter files*

These security parameters as well as all the residual risk management actions proposed in the case of this comprehensive analysis have two purposes:

– *On the device*:

    - to guarantee the user's security;

    - to guarantee the reliability of the connected non-contact thermometer;

    - to guarantee proper patient care.

– *On the users' personal health data*:

    - to guarantee the respect of the users' private lives;

    - to guarantee the respect of and access to the data.

Comprehensive Approach

8.1. Contribution from the comprehensive risk analysis process

The comprehensive risk analysis allowed us to observe that the dangers "client", "image", "information system" and "physicochemical" require a prioritization of risk-reduction actions. The "measuring the temperature" phase requires prioritization. Throughout the system, the cost of treatment is greater than the cost without treatment. It is therefore a political risk treatment. To limit the comprehensive risk analysis, the work group immediately excluded certain dangers.

Seventy-six dangerous situations with priority level 1 converted into 151 accident scenarios came out of our dangerous situation cartography, which shows that the fragilities are spread across all the retained dangers from our study. The following subfunctions, "measuring the temperature" and "sharing these measurement data with a health professional", contain more of the dangerous situations, respectively, than the subfunction "visualizing the measurements on the application", which accrues slightly fewer C3 risks than the former category. Phase C, "sharing these health data with a health professional", is the one that accumulates the least.

The reduction actions essentially concern four sections:

– reinforcing the internal clients' sound system;

– securing or protecting the application's information system;

– educating personnel;

– optimizing the thermometer sensor's decisional algorithms to improve the reliability of measurements.

At the level of the industrial actors, these actions should be progressively implemented. Certain actions like making new quick steps available to users and taking into consideration the aspect of application or software use and educating personnel on the external after-sales service to work together with the development team will be performed by the marketing team. Other actions like the implementation of a certification procedure for exchanges with the post office protocols and a protocol that allows malicious attacks to be simulated in order to identify the vulnerabilities present in the software will be performed by the mobile application managers.

8.2. New health challenges: risks emerging from the use of connected medical devices

In general, this comprehensive analysis of the risks linked to the use of connected non-contact thermometers allowed us to observe that new connected medical devices bring new practices and new solutions to preexisting problems. During the first ebola crisis, if we imagine that the populations had access to connected non-contact thermometers, this would certainly have limited the disease's contamination rate. During this same crisis, the health authorities complained about the absence of epidemiological data on multiple occasions and yet this problem could have been solved by connected non-contact thermometers.

Although these new solutions bring numerous advantages and benefits, the new risks are not to be forgotten and like the solutions given, they are innovative. Among the fears concerning these new practices in the field of healthcare, we have: the intrusion of a malicious actor in the application's database, the total or partial compromise of the application's server, the spread of a virus through a malicious file, identity theft, data piracy, cybercriminality, not to forget the danger in terms of image for the manufacturer who puts an innovation of this stature on the market when certain waves of negative opinions potentially consider their offer not to respond to the public's expectations.

We observe that the non-negligible emerging risk factors are for the most part tied to the security of the application's information system, to the brand image of the innovative company and to the reliability and use of the sensors on the proposed devices. They particularly concern the following:

– *Data confidentiality*: Intrusion of a malicious actor; private life endangered.

This concerns preventing the unauthorized spread of data. These must only be accessible by authorized entities. Although the sale of the connected non-contact thermometer seems to present a certain incompatibility with the desire to protect one's intimacy, article 226-22 of the French penal code, for example, establishes a punishment of 5 years imprisonment and a 30,000 euro fine for a person who has collected private data "whose spread would result in harm being done to the concerned party's interests or the intimacy of his or her private life, [the fact of] possessing the concerned party's data without authorization and with the knowledge of a third party without permission to receive them". Furthermore, certain manufacturers propose connected non-contact thermometers allowing geolocalization of health actors. We turn our attention toward the fact that, even if a manufacturer proposes free hosting to users within a personal health data host, the risk of intrusion remains and persists when the user chooses to share his or her data.

– *Integrity*: Pirating, identity theft, total or partial compromise of a server, intrusion of a malicious file to falsify the application's queries.

This concerns the prevention of the unauthorized modification of data. There is a non-negligible risk that malicious actors enter the database of the connected medical device's application without invitation to misappropriate information relevant to the users' sensitive data. It is also not unthinkable for hackers to insert viruses or a malicious file in the application via e-mail, for example, either with the goal to falsify the application's queries to unsettle a user or to discredit the device's manufacturer. Incidentally, risk-reduction actions have been proposed in this framework.

The ability concerning this covers the prevention of unauthorized withholding of data. Sometimes integrity can be a prerequisite for confidentiality.

– *Reinforcement of legislation*: Absence of extraterritorial laws on the collection of data via a connected medical device.

In the scope of using a connected medical device, in this case, a connected non-contact thermometer with this status, questions persist concerning the sanctions to be implemented. In relation to the volume of data collected by the product and risks linked to insecurity (illegitimate access, identity theft, viral attack, data leak, insecure Bluetooth network, impossible restoration of data, violation of professional secrecy, flaws linked to the duration of personal data conservation, etc.), a reevaluation of the legal penalties would be necessary to discourage certain malicious actors.

– *Image and the client*: Bad reputation, waves of negative opinions concerning the proposed technology.

Additionally, the image risk, in other words, everything that can harm the development of the manufacturer's current activity; a considerable number of vulnerabilities. This shows that developers should constantly improve measures that can allow them to better target the expectations of their clients and respect the quality of compatibility of their products.

PART 3

Connected Objects, a New Era for
Scientific Revolution

9

Prospects in Health

9.1. Connected medical devices, participatory contribution to research

Connected objects in healthcare will henceforth play a role in medical research issues that must be clarified.

9.1.1. *Sorting rare pathologies at the border: the case of ebola*

The hunt for emerging viruses, notably in the case of Ebola, keeps dozens of international researchers and their local partners busy in several African countries. In Europe, it has inspired the implementation of preparation plans like passenger sorting at airports and drafted role games that aim to test the state's reaction to a pandemic in the presence of health authorities.

It is in this spirit that certain manufacturers propose a technical solution to the battle against the Ebola virus: connected non-contact thermometers. This consists of sorting people along borders by measuring their temperature remotely, without contact. The data are then returned to the thermometer and transmitted via Bluetooth or Wi-Fi to the application situated in the mobile terminal, the end goal being to identify febrile individuals to avoid the contamination of the populace.

NOTE.– The company Withings has released a new health device onto the market: the Thermo, a connected non-contact thermometer that measures the temperature at the temporal artery. Data recording is therefore frontal and contact free.

These connected non-contact thermometers are really connected medical devices. The data gathered are transmitted to the health authorities and they allow for a new epidemiological approach. They reinforce the efficacy of sorting the spread of information to field workers (e-training on a tablet) and the ability to react in the face of the spread of the ebola virus.

9.2. Epidemiological monitoring

With the rise of new information technologies, connected health is developing as a consequence. Numerous clients are equipped with connected health objects such as smart scales, connected non-contact thermometers, blood pressure monitors, heart rate monitors and many others. Individuals' sensitive data are absolutely confidential because organizations like the CNIL recommend that personal data hosts take the necessary measures to ensure the confidentiality and protection of the data they are entrusted with, such as protection procedures, securing data storage devices and information system maintenance.

That said, these anonymous sensitive data will be correlated and analyzed to better follow the health situation in a country. In terms of medical research, they could also offer the possibility of following a population, to compare it with a control population, and of further research in order to make significant improvements concerning prevention and therapeutic care.

9.3. The patient becomes an active member of the healthcare team

At this point, several observations stand out:

– the days of patients waiting for a diagnosis from their doctors is now long gone. Because of advances in new technologies that facilitate access to information sources, many want to know about these and get involved in their care;

– the patient is considered the client of the hospital that expects care to come from the health team. Otherwise, if treatment is to be pursued while the patient is at home, the health team is no longer present;

– the process of harvesting a patient's health data, particularly during hospitalization, is generally very long because the health professional has several appointments on their agenda. Furthermore, the medical devices used are sometimes difficult to carry, and patient follow-up after discharge proves practically impossible. In most cases, patients suffering chronic diseases are monitored from time to time.

The introduction of connected health into patient care will allow for daily patient follow-up thanks to medical devices connected to a database. Connected health thus allows care to be made more accessible, bilateral communication between the health professional and the patient to be offered, and the public to be educated.

Health professionals are responsible for capturing data, analyzing them, establishing a diagnosis and healing the patient. Through the use of connected medical devices, patients can provide their daily data for their treatment. These are generally focused on health indicators (weight, heart rate, blood pressure, SpO_2, blood sugar, etc.).

Provided over a long period of time, these health data will allow health professionals to better predict, prevent and cure diseases via decisional algorithms incorporated into these connected devices. The patient thus becomes an actor included in the healthcare team.

9.4. Development of online portals (patient portal) with or without subscriptions

Another use of connected health objects aims to develop patient portals in order to provide interfaces offering access to online platforms coordinated by professionals. Such portals would allow them to organize the patient's health pathway. The patient will thus have access to a useful portal to:

– record data relative to follow-up, e.g. temperature, weight, pain and the observation of treatments;

– visualize and record all of their medical appointments on a calendar;

– have access to a directory with the contact information of professionals involved in their care, as well as useful phone numbers;

– directly access preselected web pages giving certified information on the disease, treatments and side effects;

– have access to a storage space to upload, archive and classify the documents relative to care (test results or measurements, medical information, performance indicators, etc.).

Doudoucare is a platform monitored by pediatric nurses. The service proposes personalized responses to parents' questions within 2 h. The questions relate to early childhood.

10

A Step Towards the Augmented Human

10.1. Transhumanism

The concept of the augmented human harks back to the transhumanist movement. To address this section, I visited the Website[1] Humanity+, the world transhumanist association. This represents a movement whose reflection is based on technique and new technologies. Transhumanists believe that the flood of nanotechnologies, biotechnologies, information and communication technologies, and cognitive science (NBIC) technologies is going to modify and improve (even expand) human potential at the physical and cognitive levels.

Now let us move on to the meaning of NBIC to better understand the meaning of this movement.

Nanotechnologies can be defined as all technology manipulating structures (electronic, chemical, etc.), devices and material systems on a nanometer (nm) scale, the equivalent of 20 hydrogen atoms. As a comparison, when put side-by-side, molecules can be several nanometers long.

The benefits of nanotechnologies can be found in diagnosis, and nanoelements allow for:

– improved performances: sensitivity, detection threshold, speed;

---

1 Association created by Swedish philosopher Nick Bostrom in 1998. Today, he teaches at Oxford University and deals with the technological risks and dangers that could be detrimental to mankind.

– the reliability and precision of results;

– the miniaturization of devices.

Likewise, in the field of therapy, the contributions of nanotechnology allow for:

– the rapid detection of pathologies;

– the improved efficacy of medications;

– the reduction of side effects and toxicity;

– the reduction of the number of active molecules;

– the increase in biocompatibility with tissue engineering.

Furthermore, the European Technology Platform Nanomedicine was created in 2006 under the auspices of the European Commission and in partnership with numerous industrial and academic actors. This platform was established in Paris within the *Ecole supérieure de physique et de chimie* (ESPCI Paris Tech) atop the Montagne Sainte-Geneviève. One of its objectives is to encourage strategic reflection and endorse the industrial and public health potential of nanomedicine to the national and European authorities. It facilitates innovation by producing strategic sector development plans.

As for biotechnology, this is all of the methods and processes arising from microbiology, biochemistry, biophysics, genetics[2], computer science, etc., to produce goods and services. The applications of biotechnology concern three primary domains: agriculture, health and industry.

With regard to agriculture, biotechnologies allow yields to be improved, for example corn resistant to the corn borer[3]. In the field of healthcare, they allow for the production of antibiotics and therapeutic proteins for genetic engineering, e.g. insulin. For industry, they offer waste water treatment techniques, for instance.

Established and emerging information and communication technologies include the techniques used in the processing and transmission of information

---

2 Discipline in biology that studies heredity.
3 Species of insect from Europe.

(audiovisual, multimedia, etc.), Internet and telecommunications. These technologies allow users to communicate, access information sources, and store and transfer information in any format (interface, video, image, texts, etc.).

10.2. The augmented human

In 1941, Julian Huxley used the word "transhumanism" for the first time. Its objective is to improve the physical and mental performance of a human through NBIC; we are speaking here of the augmented human.

A human being is not augmented because he wears optical glasses to overcome myopia. The augmentation in question aims to give man greater (travel) speed, more memory and more endurance when performing a particularly demanding task, maybe one that is even impossible at a physical, intellectual or emotional level, as well as greater resistance to physical trauma, all while maintaining good health. Here, it is important to differentiate between augmented and repaired.

> "One is not augmented by wearing a hearing aid[4] or a hip prosthesis. At this point, we are speaking of a repaired human who benefits from technology allowing him to become a valid man". Michel Besnier, panel discussion, Scientific Days at the University of Nantes, July 4, 2016.

Given that transhumanist theory is very recent, it is a scientific advancement that must still be developed in our society. This augmentation will have three principal advantages: bodily emancipation, improved physical and mental performances, and the ability to live with robots.

A human being could see several meters further than normal, he would be sensitive to infrared waves, could hear ultrasound frequencies and have the olfactory capacities of a dog to track human scents.

Given that transhumanism depends on technologies that can greatly modify our daily lives, some have already been applied without notice. Below are some examples.

---

4 Device for the hard of hearing to combat deafness. It is made up of an amplifier that is placed on the ear.

10.3. Some applications of connected health and nanotechnologies to move toward the augmented human

The rise of new information and communication technologies astounds numerous manufacturers specializing in automotives, health, environment, banking, business, energy, transport, etc. In the framework of medicine, the applications of connected e-health objects are multiplying; most of them are implemented to facilitate the emergence of the augmented human. To augment the human, transhumanists imagine starting with genetic manipulation through the implant of electronic chips in the brain. The appearance of some applications shows us this today.

EXAMPLE 10.1.– Artificial intelligence for health

Artificial intelligence algorithms are primarily based on learning. They learn to use megadata collected to then perform a task. For example, by providing millions of facial images to an algorithm, it can learn to recognize this person from among a hundred people.

Google's connected contact lenses injected directly into the eye: A patent unveiled by Forbes[5], it is a matter of injecting a contact lens directly into the eyeball. It solidifies and attaches itself to the eye with the aim of improving vision, but also to connect the wearer to a GPS, the Internet or a smartphone via wireless connection. It contains storage, sensors, a cellular chip and a battery. This battery is recharged by the user himself via a special antenna. It will display the route from a GPS in the field of vision and take photos by blinking. Connected to an adapted application, it will allow facial recognition. In terms of health, Google's connected contact lenses could also help people with presbyopia, i.e. those who cannot read without glasses.

Nanorobots could be useful in medicine, locating and destroying cancer cells. Theoretically, biorobots placed in the human body could stimulate certain nerves, or hypercomplex, multifunctional nanomachines could allow for the reconstruction of living tissues through a simple subcutaneous injection. These nanorobots, small enough to enter a living cell, could replace or locate organelles, modify nucleic acids and thus the genetic code, or perform other tasks that are impossible without invasive microsurgery. It is also imaginable for nanorobots to be able to cure cancers by destroying

---

5 https://www.forbes.com/sites/aarontilley/2016/04/28/google-device-eyeball/#361740c67201.

degenerating cells. Another possible application would be to detect toxic chemicals in the environment and to measure their concentration.

Biochips or DNA chips: their use has seen growing momentum, particularly in the field of oncology to type tumors according to their genetic profile, to compare healthy tissues with diseased tissues, treated vs. untreated, etc. It is possible to estimate the appearance of more than 30,000 genes.

EXAMPLE 10.2.– When health merges with fashion

Several projects have appeared in the fashion and health sector aiming to improve Man's physical and cognitive performances. Spanish artists Maria Castellanos and Alberto Valverde have developed a connected dress that uses several sensors to detect invisible environmental factors such as temperature, atmospheric pressure, sound or dust levels. An application is installed in the user's mobile terminal. This warns the user in the case of air contamination. In the case of noise pollution in a specific area, the user can order the application to close the helmet that is integrated into the robe to shelter the user from the noise.

The climate dress is made up of conductive embroidery, composed of 100 minuscule luminous diodes, a carbon dioxide (CO_2) detector and microprocessors developed to be integrated into a fabric. This climate dress lights up and changes the rhythm of its pulsations based on the level of CO_2 in the air, which allows the person wearing it and those around the person to measure the concentration of carbon dioxide in the air and to be aware of environmental problems.

Fashion-tech designer Anouk Wipprecht[6], creator of the spider dress, proposes a unicorn wearable headset to help children suffering from ADHD (attention deficit/hyperactivity disorder). This headset films the moments that capture the child's attention to make these recognizable and to give the child autonomy in handling this disorder.

Australian Lucy McRae is a hybrid and polymorphic artist, a body architect and she has worked with many companies. In collaboration with Philips, she created clothing that reflects a person's mood.

---

6 Source: https://iq.intel.com/unicorn-wearable-uses-neuroscience-to-help-kids/.

EXAMPLE 10.3.– Virtual reality to improve patients' care pathway at the hospital

A stay at the hospital quickly becomes long and very boring. Virtual reality headsets allow patients to escape the hospital environment. The patient is transported into very immersive fantasy worlds. This activity can have negative repercussions for the patient, but also veritable health benefits.

Bliss is an interactive 3D application that allows people in an isolated or stressful situation to escape to a virtual world. Patient morale is an important factor in recovery and after having been tested in a hospital environment, it has proven its positive effects on patients' psychological state.

The creator of this application, who develops it in collaboration with research centers, says,

"This idea is inspired by my personal experience assisting my companion during his hospitalization in a sterile room for several weeks for his leukemia treatment – a bone marrow transplant. The hospitalized person in a sterile environment lives in an extreme solitary confinement for weeks, she/he cannot put a foot down and only one member of the family has the permission to go behind the canopy after dressing up with two layers of clothing, a hygiene cap and a mask" (Mélanie Péron)[7].

These kinds of applications are truly educational tools. They allow health professionals and patients' family members to put themselves in the patients' place to understand their difficulties and better support them.

---

7 https://www.kisskissbankbank.com/bliss.

PART 4

Methodological Approach

Functional Need Analysis

11.1. Functional need analysis

The life cycle of a system most often starts with a need analysis. This allows the expected functions of services and those generated by product use to be characterized. This phase involves a whole array of activities (application of an octopus diagram, function validation, product characterization, etc.) that are also called upstream studies. This phase is an integral part of our comprehensive risk analysis process.

11.1.1. *Definition of the octopus diagram*

This is a functional analysis tool that identifies the functions of a system and researches the expected functions and their relations. All of this is done synthetically through a schema.

The infrared non-contact thermometers that are the object of our study are placed at the middle of the octopus. They are service generators between the product and the outside elements.

Next, it is a matter of describing the existing relations defining the object of the study with or between the elements from the outside. Lines connecting two elements from the outside via the connected non-contact thermometer's functioning as intermediary define the primary functions that represent a goal to be attained for the object of our study. An arrow linking an outside element represents a constraint function, which is a developmental demand.

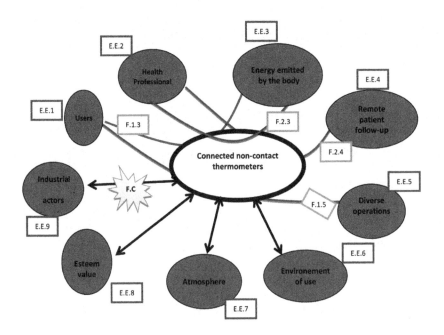

Figure 11.1. *Octopus diagram*

11.1.2. *Function validation*

This stage consists of inventorying the different functions in interaction with the outside elements. This process was performed based on connected non-contact thermometers demonstrating the characteristics found in Table 11.1.

		Validity check		Stability check	
Function between outside elements	Definition of the function	Why?	For what?	What could make this need evolve over time?	What could make it disappear over time?
All kinds of users – energy emitted	F.2.4 Measuring the body temperature remotely using the energy it emits	Having a medical device that measures the body temperature: non-invasively, with a simple, quick and ergonomic use	Monitoring the evolution of a body's temperature Defining temperature anomalies	Improving the analysis algorithm that allows the exact value of the temperature to be displayed.	Abandoning connected non-contact (infrared) technology Evolution of norms Excessive increase in acquisition prices

				Developing thermometers with a narrower viewing angle that could recognize the mode and kind of temperature measurement (forehead, ear, etc.)	Evolution of norms on the confidentiality of users' personal data
Health professionals – remote patient checkup and follow-up	F.3.5 Providing information and a checkup remotely because of data collected by the application, particularly temperature measurement data	To ensure better remote patient care. Improving practices linked to telemedicine (teleconsultation, tele-expertise, telesurveillance, etc.).	Detecting and defining difficult pathologies thanks to statistical data from the collected temperatures. Improving medical research	Conducting clinical assays to demonstrate the product's quality and precision. Offering complete education to users on mastering computer networks and telecoms (terminals, mobile networks, Internet, data center, cloud computing)	Abandoning connected non-contact (infrared) technology Abandoning connected non-contact (infrared) technology
Users – surface temperature, ambient temperature	F.2.6 Measuring the ambient temperature, Measuring the temperature of a precise surface	Having a medical device that measures temperature and that is simple, quick, and ergonomic to use	Monitoring the evolution of the temperature of a surface, electrical circuit, etc.; Knowing the temperature of a chemical;	Evolution of norms, reducing acquisition prices of the device on the market	Abandoning non-contact technology
Users – diverse and varied operations	F.2.7 Collecting temperature measurement data to gather information that is generally difficult to capture	Having a medical device that measures the body temperature: non-invasively, with a simple, quick, and ergonomic use	Monitoring the evolution of the body's temperature	Reduction of acquisition prices of the product; Associating the sale of the thermometer with that of the cell phone best suited to the application	

Table 11.1. *Validation of the functions*

11.1.3. *Product characterization*

The functional analysis allows a characterization to be made up of the service or constraint functions:

– criterion: parameter checked to appreciate the manner in which a function is fulfilled or a constraint respected;

– level: point of reference on the scale adopted for a function appreciation criterion;

– flexibility: tolerance set to indicate the possibilities of adjusting a level for a particular criterion.

This process was performed based on connected non-contact thermometers that present the characteristics found in Table 11.2.

Function	Appreciation criteria	Nominal level	Acceptance levels
Measuring the body's temperature remotely using the energy it emits	Nature: Temporal temperature; frontal temperature Temperature range: Status indication Display time Display resolution Distance focalization: Device body Vision angle: Simplicity of reading:	°C or °F (Fahrenheit) Lithium battery symbol Plus or minus 0.1 °C Plus or minus "3–5 cm", all depending on the manufacturer Plus or minus 60°–80°, all depending on the manufacturer Limited information Easy to interpret	[30–43 °C]; [86–109°F]; (Fahrenheit-32) × 5/9 = °C Recharge every 6 months (Fahrenheit-32) × 5/9 = °C, all depending on the manufacturer Plus or minus [0.1– 0.3 °C], all depending on the manufacturer Plus or minus, "3–5 cm", all depending on the manufacturer Plus or minus 60°–80°, all depending on the manufacturer No to the playback screen's saturation
Providing patients with information and a remote checkup	Monitoring patients Diagnostic aid The application's internal memory capacity	Patient or family consent to the process	Following the process over time
Measuring the ambient temperature or that of a precise surface	Nature: Ambient temperature; surface temperature Temperature range: Status indicator Display time Maximum startup Automatic stop Consumption	Example: [0–93.3 °C]; [32–199.9°F] 2 s 1 s 4 s	Example: [2–3] s [1–3] s 5 s <50 mV

Collecting measurement data to recover and analyze information that is generally difficult to capture	The data collected and provided by the application must be: - coherent, credible, exact, and pertinent. They must match the person's physical conditions The application's internal memory capacity The cell phone's internal memory capacity	User consent; Taking into consideration the application and cell phone's internal memory	Following the process over time; permanent application update

Table 11.2. *Characterization of the product*

Then, we move on to the final stage of our analysis, which is the application of the appreciation criteria for connected non-contact thermometers.

11.1.4. Appreciation criteria

At this point, it is a question of providing information presented in Table 11.3.[1]

Functions	Measuring the body's temperature remotely using the energy it emits	Ensuring a remote checkup on patients	Measuring the ambient temperature or that of a precise surface	Collecting measurement data to improve personalized care provision
Norms, regulations	ISO 14985, ISO 17025 NF EN 60721-3-2 class 2M3: 1997, shock and vibration resistant; NF EN 60950-1: 2006, security for using technological equipment; NF EN 50082-1: 1998 electromagnetic sensitivity: demands relative to immunity against electromagnetic disturbances for electric and electronic devices Directive 98/37/CE from June 22, 1998, concerning the comparison of member states' legislation relative to the guarantee of the highest level security possible	Article 7 of EITL	ISO 14985; NF EN 60721-3-2 classes 2M3: 1997; NF EN 60950-1: 2006; NF EN 50082-1: 1998; Directive 98/37/CE from June 22, 1998	Federal law on data protection Article 49 of the Public Market Code (on tests of samples) Article 323-1 of penal code L.1111-8 from the Public Health Code from law no. 2002-303

---

1 All legal guidelines mentioned in the table below are from French legal texts.

Level of ergonomics, implementation	Weight, dimension, grip, cable Transport system: Base, carrying case Power supply: USB port, universal charger; rechargeable batteries	Data management: Transmission and recording through the application installed on the mobile terminal On-screen indicators: Personalizable screen; powering up	Weight Dimension Grip	
Level of comfort	Resisting high temperatures, resisting shock; black-on-white display screen for the thermometer; portable device		Resisting high temperatures, resisting shock	
Adaptation to use	Wet environment. Partial or total darkness; change in screen color based on temperature level; Low enough mass to measuring the temperature easily; rather limited number of buttons on the device		Surface limits: Not all surfaces have the same emissivity (ε) (ε) of asbestos = 0.95 (ε) of limestone = 0.98 (ε) of soil = 0.92–0.96 (ε) of sand = 0.90	
Lifetime, sustainability, solidity	Replacement battery available; charge time responds to operational use as best possible			
Level of functional security	Warnings when exceeding maximum use temperature (audio or visual signal)			

Table 11.3. *Appreciation of criteria*

Comprehensive Risk Scenario Analysis Cartography

12.1. Method

After having established the dangerous situation cartography and determining the different evaluation scales, we ascertained several scenarios. From this we deduced a feared event that can be associated with each priority 1 dangerous situation.

The accident scenarios were obtained in the following way:

– the convergence of a danger (or dangerous element) and a contact event;

– a dangerous situation confronted by the occurrence of a primer event creates a feared event or accident for which the gravity of all consequences is determined.

Table 12.1 presents our risk scenario analysis cartography. The final column corresponds to the management of residual risk.

Dangerous situation	Contact causes	Feared event	Primer causes	Already existing treatments including means of detection or alert	Consequences	Gi	Li	Ci	IP	Risk-reduction actions and identification of the deciding authority for their application	RRM
Non-application of the norms relative to the processing of data with a connected object	Extraterritorial divergences concerning regulation	Legal penalties	*Audit performed by the competent authority*	NO	13 Warning without formal notice followed by an offer for free regularization	1	2	1			
Failures with respect to the norms relative to the processing of data with a connected medical device	Regulation linked to the use of connected devices	Legal penalties	*Audit performed by the competent authority*	NO	13 Warning without formal notice followed by an offer for free regularization	1	3		1		
Failures with respect to norms	Regulation linked to the use of connected devices	Complaints and claims from third parties	*Audit performed by the competent authority*	NO	23 Orders to stop processing litigious data	2	3		1		
Alteration of the device's physical integrity	Exposal of the device to conditions that are incompatible with its operating instructions	Inability to take a temperature reading	*Need to perform a remote temperature reading*	Informative tables given to the client upon purchase of the device. They give explanations of: -operating instructions -measurement -safety recommendations -warnings before first use of the functions	14 Client dissatisfaction without claims	1			1		
Pollution	Presence of combustible products	Total alteration of the temperature data's physical integrity	*Remote temperature reading with the device*	Informative tables given to the client upon purchase of the device. They give explanations of: -operating instructions -measurement -safety recommendations -warnings before first use of the functions	31 Unavailability of the device <10 min + consequent data alteration	1		3	1		

Risk	Cause	Effect	Need	Measures / Protocols	Consequence			
Technology ill-adapted to the presence of external electromagnetic fields	Presence of an electric or magnetic source (television, microwave oven)	Inability to obtain reliable temperature data	*Need to perform a remote temperature reading with the device*	Informative tables given to the client upon purchase of the device. They give explanations of: -operating instructions -measurement -safety recommendations -warnings before first use of the functions	14 Client dissatisfaction without claims	1	2	1
Erroneous data	Difficulty using the device or taking a temperature reading	Therapeutic error	*Electronic transmission of the obtained health data to a health professional for remote care*	NO	13 Warning without formal notice followed by an offer for free regularization	1	2	1
Inability to respect the measurement distance	Absence of a health professional to arrange the remote temperature reading on the patient	Contamination of the vicinity	*Ill user*	Education of distributors and buyers on available paper, electronic, and online video products.	54 Permanent disability or death	5		1
Inability of the patient to connect to the application	Incorrect entry protocol after intrusion by a malicious actor	Inability to supply the health database to conduct research on difficult pathologies	*Need to transmit data for medical research centers*	Implementation of the following protocols: 1-FIREWALL that allows access to the server port to be blocked. 2- Level 7 FIREWALL that allows the presence of viruses in the software layer to be detected.	14 Client dissatisfaction without claims	1	2	1
Obtention of corrupted data (lost, altered)	Injection of a malicious file	Inability to provide remote care	*Need to transfer data for a prescription or remote care*	Server analysis and data reintegration if necessary. Storage on virtual servers with multiple backups on multiple sites. Regular backups in multiple locations.	42 Recovery or correction of the data with a consequent financial loss < 2000€	4		1

Risk	Cause	Effect	Context	Measures	Consequence				Recommended action	
Total compromise of the application's server	Injection of a malicious file	Inability to provide remote care	*Need to transmit data for remote care*	Implementation of the following protocols: 1-FIREWALL that allows access to the server port to be blocked. 2- Level 7 FIREWALL that allows the presence of viruses in the software layer to be detected.	**52 Recovery or correction of the data with a financial loss < 3000€**	5	2	2	2	A1 Drafting a protocol that allows data to be encrypted by the telephone and decrypted by the server, which alone has the key. A5 Drafting a protocol allows malicious attacks to be simulated in order to identify the vulnerabilities present in the software	
Partial alteration of the device's physical integrity	Device left within reach of children	Inability to perform a temperature reading with the thermometer	*Need to use the device*	Operating instructions Tutorial videos on website and within the application.	41 Device unavailability >10 min with partial data loss	4	1	1	2		
Pejorative *a priori* on the proposed technology (loss of credibility)	No confidence building with clients concerning the proposed technology	Drop in sales and loss of revenue	*Implementation of several device sales points*	Social network management by a provider to respond to criticism and take it into consideration. Moderate statements on networks	43 Complaint followed by a conviction and moderate restitution < 100000€	4	5	3	3	A2 Drafting an external level 1 SAV procedure that works together with the development team.	*P2*
Putting batches of defective devices on the market	Design flaws in one or multiple thermometers put on the market	Clients publicize their dissatisfaction	*Use of devices by clients*	Design qualification Product sampling procedure at warehouse Product recall procedure (catastrophic)	53 Conviction of the manufacturer with financial penalties between 100000€ and 300000€	5	3	3	2	A3 Educating personnel on (sample) quality control for products at the warehouse	

Risk	Cause	Effect	Event	Existing measures	Consequence				Recommended action
Inability to share data with a health professional	Lacking know-how in the use of computer applications	Disturbance of care	Prescription for remote care	Informative tables and quick steps produced provided to the client upon buying the device. They provide explanations on the operating instructions and measurement Video tutorials	24 Financial losses < 500€	2	3	1	A7 Making new quick steps available to users, taking into account the aspect of using the application on the mobile terminal
Scared, frightened patient	Cognitive issues, trembling, joint pain	Change of heart by a patient who totally refuses remote care	Confirmation of the patient's consent for remote care	Behavioral, cognitive, and nervous issues are reasons not to use connected objects and exclusion criteria in telehealth.	24 Financial losses < 500€	2	2	1	
Complex operation instructions	Poor product demonstration to target clients	Obtention of unreliable data due to an improper choice of measurement mode	Remote temperature reading by client	Informative tables given to the client upon purchase of the device. They give explanations of: -operating instructions -measurement -safety recommendations -warnings before first use of the functions	34 Financial losses between 500€ and 5000€	3	3	2	A13 Promoting the education of pharmacists or health professionals concerning telehealth and/or telemedicine
Inability to transmit data to the health professional	Lacking mastery of new information technologies	Data-transmission service not provided or not possible, leading to disturbance in care	Need to transmit data for remote care	Informative tables and quick steps produced provided to the client upon buying the device. They provide explanations on the operating instructions and measurement	34 Financial losses between 500€ and 5000€	3	3	2	A7 Making new quick steps available to users, taking into account the aspect of using the application on the mobile terminal

Risk	Cause	Consequence	Event	Existing measures	Criticality				Actions
Inability to transmit data	Lacking mastery of new information technologies	Inability to provide the health database allowing research to be performed on difficult pathologies	*Confirmation of the patient's consent to medical research using his or her health data*	Informative tables are provided to the client upon buying the device. They provide explanations on the operating instructions and measurement	34 Financial losses between 500€ and 5000€	3	3	2	2	A7 Making new quick steps available to users, taking into account the aspect of using the application on the mobile terminal
Creation of the patient file by a replacement doctor who is unaware of telemedicine and/or telehealth	Unavailability of the health professional following a change in planning	Issuance of an ambiguous, confusing, and/or contradictory diagnosis	*Analysis of the health file by the health professional*	NO	24 Financial losses < 500€	2		1	1	
Non-compliant devices put on the market	Tools not appropriate for the ensurance of device quality control	Financial loss, loss of brand confidence and credibility	*Purchase + use of devices*	Development qualification compliant with good medical device production practices in the factory. Sampling procedure in the warehouse	43 Complaint followed by a conviction and moderate restitution < 100000€	4		2	2	3	A3 Educating personnel on (sample) quality control for products at the warehouse.
Management of non-conformities is performed by an unauthorized person	Lack of qualified, competent personnel in the domain	Legal penalties (amends and sentences), market recall (ban on sales, updated product standards)	*Complaint filed by the patient, by a competitor, by a client*	The responsible administrative and financial party performs the necessary verifications (sometimes a posteriori), subcontracting to an external company to verify regulatory elements	44 Financial loss + damages and interest between 5000€ and 100000€	4		2	2	A17 Implementing a product launch procedure with all the elements necessary for the launch. A3 Educating personnel on (sample) quality control for products at the warehouse

Event	Cause	Consequence	Description	Scenario	Impact					Action
Obsolete version put on the market	Absence of protocols on updates installed on the application	Legal penalties	The update replaces the preceding version. The only way for an outdated version to be on a smartphone is if the person has not installed the update. For major updates, information is saved for several months to give users time to install the update.	*Performance of an a posteriori check on the application on the mobile terminal*	33 Withdrawn authorization or lockout (by the CNIL) of data + amends < 3000€	3	3	2	2	A4 Making information campaign forms available to users by email to notify them about critical updates.
Inability to use the application on the mobile terminal	Unavailability of certain application functionalities	Inability to perform remote care	Implementation of a log-verification protocol in case of errors.	*Prescription requiring a transfer of personal data for remote care*	51 Total unavailability of the device, failure of service	5	2	2	2	A5 Drafting a protocol allows malicious attacks to be simulated in order to identify the vulnerabilities present in the software
Inability to use the application on the mobile terminal	Unavailability of certain application functionalities	Inability to perform remote care	Implementation of a log-verification protocol in case of errors.	*Need to transfer data to medical research centers*	51 Total unavailability of the device, failure of service	5	1	1		
Failure to keep the patient's sensitive data	Application access rights are less or badly protected	Voluntary disclosure of data by a malicious actor	Implementation of the following protocols: 1-FIREWALL that allows access to the server port to be blocked. 2- Level 7 FIREWALL that allows the presence of viruses in the software layer to be detected.	*Electronic transmission of data to provide remote care*	42 Recovery or correction of the data with a consequent financial loss < 2000€	4	2	2	2	A1 Drafting a protocol that allows data to be encrypted by the telephone and decrypted by the server, which alone has the key. A14 Implementing a strong identification protocol to protect access to the database (for health professionals).

Risk	Cause	Sanction	Control	Measure	Consequence		
Patient refusal to transmit data	Absence of informed and written patient consent on the management of his or her data	Aggressive speech by the health professional towards the patient	Irritation of the health professional	Patient excluded from the fact of not having signed the informed consent form.	13 Warning without formal notice followed by an offer for free regularization	1	1
Failure to respect regulations	Putting a defective connected medical device on the market	Civil and punitive sanction	*Investigation performed by competent authorities*	Obtention of the CE mark, medical class IIa, and FDA for the object + application	23 Orders to stop processing litigious data	2	1
Fraudulent data use	Non-anonymization of the data to be processed (by the host)	Civil and punitive sanction	*Investigation performed by competent authorities*	Implementation of the FHIR data format. C is a data format adapted to the medical domain. The sent medical data are separated from the patient's identity. Within the BDB, there is no direct link between the patient and his or her data. Due to this fact, it is more complicated to reassociate captured data to a patient identity or profile.	53 Conviction of the manufacturer with financial penalties between 100000€ and 300000€	5	1
Duration of data conservation exceeded	Regulatory constraints	Civil and punitive sanction	*Investigation performed by competent authorities*	Obligation to guarantee data hosting for a duration of 10 years (HSDS)	23 Orders to stop processing litigious data	2	1
Improper health data processing	Lack of respect for patient rights	Civil and punitive sanction on the host	*Complaint filed by the patient*	Patient's informed consent	43 Complaint followed by a conviction and moderate restitution < 100000€	4	1
Over and/or overestimation of acquisition costs	Presence of similar technology with more affordable acquisition prices	Failure to reach fixed sales goals and reduced profits	*Release of devices on the market*	Competition and technology monitoring	14 Client dissatisfaction without claims	1	3

Risk	Cause	Consequence	Need / Reason	Existing measures	Impact			
Improper estimation of maintenance costs	Veritable absence of competitive maintenance prices	Loss of market shares	*Purchase of devices by clients*	NO	14 Client dissatisfaction without claims	1	3	1
Improper estimation of guarantees (in terms of cost and life)	Veritable absence of competitive guarantee prices	Total or partial loss of market shares	*Purchase of devices by clients*	Conformity with the applicable regulations with a minimum 2-year guarantee.	24 Financial losses < 500€	2	1	1
Inability to make the device work	Device not fed with data	Inability to monitor temperature readings	*Need to follow the temperature*	Informative tables given to the client upon purchase of the device. They give explanations of: -operating instructions -measurement -safety recommendations -warnings before first use of the functions	11 Unavailability of the device <5 min without measure data alteration	1	2	1
Damaged device	Strong electric discharge after a surge	Inability to take a temperature reading	*Need to use the device for temperature monitoring*	NO	51 Total unavailability of the device, failure of service	5	1	1
Damaged device	Strong electric discharge after a surge	Inability to take a temperature reading	*Need to use the device for temperature monitoring*	NO	14 Client dissatisfaction without claims	1	1	1
Damaged device	Strong electric discharge after a surge	Inability to use the device and inability to feed the database for research on difficult pathologies	*Need to transmit data to feed medical research centers*	NO	14 Client dissatisfaction without claims	1	1	1
Inability to access data	Exponential increase in the flow of data transmitted by users	Saturation of storage units	*The users' desire to always have more data, for better follow-up*	Storage on virtual servers with multiple safeguards on multiple sites In case of memory saturation, existence of a protocol that uses algorithms to search for orphan data	41 Device unavailability >10 min with partial data loss	4	1	1

Free access to users' data	Application database less or not secure		Server analysis and data reintegration if necessary.		A1 Drafting a protocol that allows data to be encrypted by the telephone and decrypted by the server, which alone has the key.			
		Modification of users' personal data by a malicious actor	Implementation of the following protocols:	Entry of a malicious actor into the application's database	A16 Drafting a certificate procedure for exchanges with the POPs.			
			1- FIREWALL that allows access to the server port to be blocked.		This will allow proper communication between 2 recognized sources to be ensured. The POPs server securely identifies the manufacturer's server and vice-versa.	4	2	2	2
			2- Level 7 FIREWALL that allows the presence of viruses in the software layer to be detected.	43 Complaint followed by a conviction and moderate restitution < 100000€	A5 Drafting a protocol allows malicious attacks to be simulated in order to identify the vulnerabilities present in the software			

Free access to users' data	Application database less or not secure	Voluntary disclosure of data to the greater public by a malicious actor	*Entry of a malicious actor into the application's database*	Server analysis and data reintegration if necessary.		A1 — Drafting a protocol that allows data to be encrypted by the telephone and decrypted by the server, which alone has the key.
				Implementation of the following protocols:	43 Complaint followed by a conviction and moderate restitution < 100000€	A16 — Drafting a certificate procedure for exchanges with the POPs. This will allow proper communication between 2 recognized sources to be ensured. The POPs server securely identifies the manufacturer's server and vice-versa.
				1-FIREWALL that allows access to the server port to be blocked.	4 2 2 2	A14 — Implementing a strong identification protocol to protect access to the database (for health professionals).
				2- Level 7 FIREWALL that allows the presence of viruses in the software layer to be detected.		A5 — Drafting a protocol allows malicious attacks to be simulated in order to identify the vulnerabilities present in the software.

Risk	Cause	Consequence	Need	Measures	Impact					Recommendation
Regular interruption of the application's functionalities	Server failure	Loss or modification of sensitive data to perform the therapeutic analysis	*Need to transmit data to a health professional*	Server analysis and data reintegration if necessary. Implementation of the following protocols: 1-FIREWALL that allows access to the server port to be blocked. 2- Level 7 FIREWALL that allows the presence of viruses in the software layer to be detected.	33 Withdrawn authorization or lockout (by the CNIL) of data + amends < 3000€	3	3	2	2	A16 Drafting a certificate procedure for exchanges with the POPs. This will allow proper communication between 2 recognized sources to be ensured. The POPs server securely identifies the manufacturer's server and vice-versa.
Access to raw data and data modification	Use of a sniffer (probe that captures raw data in the air)	Analysis error and therapeutic error	*Transmission of data to the health professional*	Server analysis and data reintegration if necessary. Implementation of the following protocols: 1-FIREWALL that allows access to the server port to be blocked. 2- Level 7 FIREWALL that allows the presence of viruses in the software layer to be detected.	54 Permanent disability or death	5	2	2	2	A5 Drafting a protocol allows malicious attacks to be simulated in order to identify the vulnerabilities present in the software

Risk	Cause	Consequence	Context	Safeguards / Protocols	Impact			
Absence of regular data safeguard protocols	Uncontrolled safeguard	Loss of sensitive data	*Use of the application to transmit or follow health data*	Server analysis and data reintegration if necessary. Storage on virtual servers with multiple safeguards on multiple sites. Regular safeguards on multiple back-ups.	43 Complaint followed by a conviction and moderate restitution < 100000€	4	1	1
				Server analysis and data reintegration if necessary. Storage on virtual servers with multiple safeguards on multiple sites. Regular safeguards on multiple back-ups.	34 Financial losses between 500€ and 5000€	3	1	1
Loss or modification of strategic data for patient follow-up	Problem connected to the systematic safeguard protocol	Error in diagnostic, analytical and therapeutic decisions	*Remote patient care*					
System contamination by a virus	Presence of a malicious file on the application	Data alteration or destruction	*Use of the application*	Implementation of the following protocols: 1-FIREWALL, that allows access to the server port to be blocked. 2- Level 7 FIREWALL that allows the presence of viruses in the software layer to be detected.	42 Recovery or correction of the data with a consequent financial loss <2000€	4	2	2
Improper application initialization instruction	Improper manipulation (improper choice of an application functionality)	Inability to read the value on the telephone	*Need to transfer data to the application*	Server analysis and data reintegration if necessary.	41 Device unavailability > 10 min with partial data loss	4	1	1

A5

Drafting a protocol allows malicious attacks to be simulated in order to identify the vulnerabilities present in the software — 1

Feared event	Cause	Consequence	Context	Safety measure	Risk scenario				Action	Ref
Falsification of application queries	Execution or intrusion of a malicious file	Total loss or modification of sensitive data	*Need to use the application on the mobile terminal to transfer health data to a professional for remote care*	Implementation of the following protocols: 1-FIREWALL that allows access to the server port to be blocked. 2- Level 7 FIREWALL that allows the presence of viruses in the software layer to be detected.	32 Data recovery or correction with major financial losses < 1000€	3	2	1		
Falsification of application queries	Third-party claims		*Free access to health data (by unauthorized people)*	Implementation of the following protocols: 1-FIREWALL that allows access to the server port to be blocked. 2- Level 7 FIREWALL that allows the presence of viruses in the software layer to be detected.						*P1 and P3*
	Execution or intrusion of a malicious file				52 Recovery or correction of the data with a financial loss < 3000€	5	3	1	A6 Drafting an automated database cleaning procedure.	
Server capacity (saturated memory) exceeded	Considerable increase in the flow of data	Loss of temperature data	*Growing desire of users to follow their health data with a connected device*	In case of memory saturation, existence of a protocol that uses algorithms to search for orphan data	41 Device unavailability > 10 mn with partial data loss	4	1			
Interruption of the application's functionalities	Technical failure	Loss of sensitive data	*Need to transmit data to a health professional for remote care*	NO	51 Total unavailability of the device, failure of service	5	2	3	A6 Drafting an automated database cleaning procedure.	

Inability to transfer data via the application on the mobile terminal	Technical failure	Inability to transmit health data for the provision of care	*Need to transfer data to the doctor for patient care*	NO	41 Device unavailability > 10 min with partial data loss	4	1	1	
Inability to transfer data via the application on the mobile terminal	Technical failure leading to temporary network unavailability	Inability to transmit health data for the provision of care	*Patient care*	NO	22 Data recovery or correction with minor financial losses < 500€	2	2	1	
Inability to transfer data via the application on the mobile terminal	Technical failure leading to temporary network unavailability	Inability to feed health databases to perform research on difficult pathologies	*Confirmation of the patient's consent on the transfer of his or her personal data to medical research centers for statistical means*	NO	14 Client dissatisfaction without claims	1	1	1	
Modification of the physical integrity of data	Cyberattack after a deliberate attempt by a malicious actor to destabilize the system	Error in a diagnostic, analytical, or therapeutic decision	*Provision of care for remote care*	Implementation of the protocol FIREWALL that allows access to the server port to be blocked.	22 Data recovery or correction with minor financial losses < 500€	2	2	1	A1 Drafting a protocol that allows data to be encrypted by the telephone and decrypted by the server, which alone has the key.
Modification of the physical integrity of data	Cyberattack after a deliberate attempt by a malicious actor to destabilize the system	Complaints and claims by third parties	*Inspections and investigations by the competent authority*	Server analysis and data reintegration if necessary. Implementation of the following protocols: 1-FIREWALL that allows access to the server port to be blocked. 2- Level 7 FIREWALL that allows the presence of viruses in the software layer to be detected.	53 Conviction of the manufacturer with financial penalties between 100000€ and 300000€	5	2	2	A5 Drafting a protocol that allows malicious attacks to be simulated in order to identify the vulnerabilities present in the software

Risk	Cause	Consequence	Situation	Action	Evaluation				Proposed action
Inability to use the proposed technology	Very complex operation instructions	Decrease in device sales on the market	*Need to use a device that takes remote temperature readings*	Informative tables given to the client upon purchase of the device. They give explanations of: -operating instructions -measurement -safety recommendations -warnings before first use of the functions	24 Financial losses < 500€	2	3	1	
Developer and client stock shortage	Poor sales forecast, delayed transport, delayed manufacturing at the factory, production time (and component supply)	Loss of clients, loss of sales revenue	*Orders placed by clients*	Implementation of a stock management procedure at the warehouse	51 Total unavailability of the device, failure of service	5	2	2	A8 Drafting a procedure to improve sales forecast management
Developer and client stock shortage	Lack of raw materials to develop certain critical components	Loss of the manufacturer's competitiveness compared to competitors	*Orders placed by clients*	Implementation of a stock management procedure at the warehouse	24 Financial losses < 500€	2	2	1	A15 Drafting an improvement procedure for the computer tool (WAVESOFT)
Putting defective devices on the market	Inexistence or ignorance of procedures aiming to ensure the quality of the thermometers	Disputes with clients	*Purchase of devices by clients*	Hiring of a person capable of managing this kind of procedure at the warehouse by educating the person currently in this position if necessary	34 Financial losses between 500€ and 5000€	3	2	1	
Perfectible device performance	Misunderstood regulation	Reduced sales	*Device use by clientele*	R&D	34 Financial losses between 500€ and 5000€	3	2	1	

Risk	Cause	Failure	Activity	Treatment	Consequence				Action
Unreliable data	Poorly defined or misunderstood technical constraints	Failure to achieve fixed sales goals	*Putting devices on the market*	R&D	43 Complaint followed by a conviction and moderate restitution < 100000€	4	3	2	A12 Evaluating the electromagnetic flow on the surface of the skin in order to improve the precision of the algorithm
Indicator management is performed by unqualified personnel	Absence of definition, implementation, and follow-up of device performance indicators	Obtention of unreliable data	*Remote temperature reading with the device*	Hiring of a person capable of managing this kind of procedure at the warehouse by educating the person currently in this position if necessary	24 Financial losses < 500€	2	2	1	
Altered brightness of LCD screens	Improperly expressed or applied service mode	Improper interpretation of measurement data	*Device use*	Informative tables given to the client upon purchase of the device. They give explanations of: -operating instructions -measurement -safety recommendations -warnings before first use of the functions	14 Client dissatisfaction without claims	1	2	1	
Illegal data use	Inexperienced health professional for participation in required care (assigned or in training)	Voluntary disclosure of data to a health professional	*Patient care*	NO	43 Complaint followed by a conviction and moderate restitution < 100000€	4	2	1	A16 Drafting a certificate procedure for exchanges with the POPs. This will allow proper communication between 2 recognized sources to be ensured. The POPs server securely identifies the manufacturer's server and vice-versa.

Self-medication	Lack of respect for the general conditions of use by the patient	Improper interpretation of the action to be taken or inappropriate advice	*Purchase of medications without a prescription*	Informative tables given to the client upon purchase of the device. They give explanations of: -operating instructions -measurement -safety recommendations -warnings before first use of the functions. The TOU explain the application's limits, notably that the application is not a substitute for a health professional	13 Warning without formal notice followed by an offer for free regularization	1	2	1
Intrusion of the application's database by an unauthorized person	Deliberate attempt by a malicious actor to destabilize the system or steal data	Sensitive data leakage	*Falsification of queries*	Implementation of the following protocols: 1-FIREWALL that allows access to the server port to be blocked. 2- Level 7 FIREWALL that allows the presence of viruses in the software layer to be detected. Detection of unexpected, if correctly identified, behavior.	43 Complaint followed by a conviction and moderate restitution <100000€	4	1	
Lack of respect for the measuring distance	Measuring temperature remotely	Obtention of unreliable data	*Need to read and interpret data*	Informative tables given to the client upon purchase of the device. They give explanations of: -operating instructions -measurement -safety recommendations -warnings before first use of the functions	14 Client dissatisfaction without claims	1	3	1

				Measures	Consequence			
Device not fed	Misunderstood operating instructions	Inability to take a temperature reading	*Need to use the device*	Informative tables given to the client upon purchase of the device. They give explanations of: -operating instructions -measurement -safety recommendations -warnings before first use of the functions	21 Unavailability of the device > 5 min with service delay but data recovery	2	2	1
Device not fed	Misunderstood operating instructions	Disturbed care	*Need to use the device*	Informative tables given to the client upon purchase of the device. They give explanations of: -operating instructions -measurement -safety recommendations -warnings before first use of the functions	24 Financial losses < 500€	2	2	1
Self-medication	Respect for regulations	Undergoing improper treatment in terms of quality or dosage	*Decision to undergo a treatment related to self-medication without medical advice for treatments excluding self-medication*	Informative tables given to the client upon purchase of the device. They give explanations of: -operating instructions -measurement -safety recommendations -warnings before first use of the functions	54 Permanent disability or death	5	1	1
Inability to connect to the application	Lost or forgotten access codes	Health professional unable to provide a diagnosis due to a lack of health data	*Need to transmit health data to the practitioner for provision of remote care*	The use of an encrypting key to alter the connection username and password, as well as certain usernames used by partners. This allows identity theft to be limited (username and password)	32 Data recovery or correction with major financial losses < 1000€	3	2	1

Inability to connect to the application	Loss of access codes	Inability to transfer data to conduct statistics on serious pathologies	*Medical research centers waiting for data*	Access code recovery procedure	1 1 Unavailability of the device <5 min without measure data alteration	1	1
Uncharged device	Power surge	Inability to take a temperature reading	*Need to use the device*	Informative tables given to the client upon purchase of the device. They give explanations of: -operating instructions -measurement -safety recommendations -warnings before first use of the functions	3 1 Unavailability of the device <10 min + consequent data alteration	3	2
Presence of reddish rust on the device	Oxidation of the device or components	Alteration of the device's physical integrity	*Device use*	Informative tables given to the client upon purchase of the device. They give explanations of: -operating instructions -measurement -safety recommendations -warnings before first use of the functions 2-year guarantee	5 1 Total unavailability of the device, failure of service	5	1
Presence of reddish rust on the device	Oxidation of the device or components	Alteration of the temperature data's physical integrity	*Device use*	Informative tables given to the client upon purchase of the device. They give explanations of: -operating instructions -measurement -safety recommendations -warnings before first use of the functions 2-year guarantee	5 1 Total unavailability of the device, failure of service	5	1

Risk	Cause	Effect	Context	Existing measures	Consequence					Actions	P
External temperature reading (temperature above 35°C)	Presence of several factors capable of influencing energy harvesting	Unreliable, corrupted data	*Reading temperature data on the digital LCD screen*	Ongoing support R&D	14 Client dissatisfaction without claims	1	3	1			
External temperature reading (temperature below 32°C)	Presence of several factors capable of influencing energy harvesting	Unreliable, corrupted data	*Reading temperature data on the digital LCD screen*	Ongoing support R&D	14 Client dissatisfaction without claims	1	3	1		A10 Implementing a system to analyze surface blood flow by camera/probe. A11 Implementing a protocol to analyze skin composition by camera.	
Improper processing loop	Improper logical calculation of the sensor's decisional algorithms	Unreliable data	*Device use*	Ongoing support R&D	43 Complaint followed by a conviction and moderate restitution < 100000€	4	5	3	2	A12 Evaluating the electromagnetic flow on the surface of the skin in order to improve the precision of the algorithm	P1
Reduced skin radiation	*Diseased skin*	Obtention of unreliable data	*Use of the device for a temperature reading*	Informative tables given to the client upon purchase of the device. They give explanations of: -operating instructions -measurement -safety recommendations -warnings before first use of the functions	14 Client dissatisfaction without claims	1	3	1			

Risk	Cause	Effect	Need	Measure	Impact				A9 — Improving the precision of infrared waves by integrating a new probe into the device.
Destruction of the device	Storage of the thermometer on multiple insecure shelves	Inability to monitor health indicators (daily temperature)	*Need to monitor health indicators*	Informative tables given to the client upon purchase of the device. They give explanations of: -operating instructions -measurement -safety recommendations -warnings before first use of the functions	51 Total unavailability of the device, failure of service	5	1	1	
Improper (data) transfer frequency	Inconsistent wait time	Inability to follow measurement data	*Need to monitor temperature data*	Implementation of indicators like the establishment of a Bluetooth connection on the screen, which allows confirmation that the connection has been established and the data transfer performed.	14 Client dissatisfaction without claims	1	2	2	
Improper data transmission loop	Improper logical calculation leading to an inconsistent response time	Inability to transmit data via the application	*Application use*	Implementation of indicators like the establishment of a Bluetooth connection on the screen, which allows confirmation that the connection has been established and the data transfer performed.	14 Client dissatisfaction without claims	1	1	1	
Improper estimation of the analog values	Improper instruction or sequence order execution	Obtention of incorrect, unreliable, corrupted data	*Need to transmit data*	NO	20 Degraded system performance with no impact on security		2	2	
Improper estimation of the analog values	Output procedure error	Obtention of incorrect, unreliable data	*Remote temperature reading*	NO	32 Data recovery or correction with major financial losses < 1000€	3	3	3	1

Scenario	Cause	Consequence	Need	Safeguards	Residual risk				A9
Improper estimation of the analog values	Probe output procedure error	Error in diagnostic, analytical, and therapeutic decisions	*Need to transmit data for remote patient care by a health professional*	NO	42 Recovery or correction of the data with a consequent financial loss < 2000€	4	2	2	2	Improving the precision of infrared waves by integrating a new probe into the device.
Obtention of corrupted (lost, altered) data	Injection of a malicious file	Error in diagnostic, analytical, and therapeutic decisions	*Reception and display of data by the health professional for care provision*	Server analysis and data reintegration if necessary. Storage on virtual servers with multiple safeguards on multiple sites. Regular safeguards on multiple back-ups.	42 Recovery or correction of the data with a consequent financial loss < 2000€	4	1		
Intrusion of the application's database by an unauthorized person	Deliberate willingness of a malicious actor to destabilize the system or steal data	Improper data treatment by the application's decisional algorithms	*Falsification of queries*	The use of an encrypting key to alter the connection username and password, as well as certain usernames used by partners. This allows identity theft to be limited (username and password) + FIREWALL	34 Financial losses between 500€ and 5000€	3	2	1	
Inability to connect to the application on the mobile terminal	Lost access codes	Patient care disturbed	*Health professional waiting for data*	Access code recovery procedure	11 Unavailability of the device <5 min without measure data alteration	1	2	1	

Failure	Cause	Effect	Need	Control	Risk					Actions	P1
Improper processing loop	Improper logical calculation	Improper data interpretation	*Device use*	Ongoing support R&D	43 Complaint followed by a conviction and moderate restitution < 100000€	4	5	3	2	A10 Drafting a system to analyze surface blood flow by camera/probe. A11 Drafting a protocol to analyze skin composition by camera. A12 Evaluating the electromagnetic flow on the surface of the skin in order to improve the precision of the algorithm.	
Alteration of the device's physical integrity	Device exposed to atmospheric conditions incompatible with its operating instructions	Inability to take a temperature reading	*Need to perform a remote temperature reading*	NO	51 Total unavailability of the device, failure of service	5	1				
Incorrect data	Difficulty using the device, taking a temperature reading	Analysis error	*Electronic transmission of health data for remote care*	Operating instructions Video tutorials on website and on the application	13 Warning without formal notice followed by an offer for free regularization	1	2	1			
Patient inability to connect to the application	Improper input protocol after intrusion by a malicious actor	Inability to feed the database with data to conduct research on difficult pathologies	*Need to transmit data for medical research centers*	Implementation of the following protocols: 1-FIREWALL that allows access to the server port to be blocked. 2- Level 7 FIREWALL that allows the presence of viruses in the software layer to be detected.	14 Client dissatisfaction without claims	1	1				

Risk	Cause	Consequence	Need	Measures	Impact				Recommendation
Total compromise of the application's server	Injection of a malicious file	Inability to make a therapeutic decision due to a lack of health data	*Need to transmit data for remote care*	Implementation of the following protocols: 1-FIREWALL that allows access to the server port to be blocked. 2- Level 7 FIREWALL that allows the presence of viruses in the software layer to be detected.	24 Financial losses < 500€	2	2	1	
Partial alteration of the device's physical integrity	Device left within reach of children	Obtention of unreliable measurement data	*Need to use the device*	Informative tables given to the client upon purchase of the device. They give explanations of: -operating instructions -measurement -safety recommendations -warnings before first use of the functions	14 Client dissatisfaction without claims	1	1	1	
Inability to transmit data to the health professional	Lacking mastery of new information technologies	Error in diagnostic, analytical, and therapeutic decisions	*Need to transmit data for remote care*	Informative tables and quick steps produced provided to the client upon buying the device. They provide explanations on the operating instructions and measurement	24 Financial losses < 500€	2	5	2	1 A16 Drafting a certificate procedure for exchanges with the POPs. This will allow proper communication between 2 recognized sources to be ensured. The POP's server securely identifies the manufacturer's server and vice-versa.

Outdated version put on the market	Absence of protocols to check for updates installed on the application	Legal penalties	*Performance of an a posteriori control on the mobile terminal by the competent authorities*	The update replaces the preceding version. The only way for an outdated version to be on a smartphone is if the person has not updated. For major updates, information is conserved for several months to leave users time to update.	21 Unavailability of the device > 5 min with service delay but data recovery	2	3
Under and/or overestimation of acquisition costs	Presence of similar technology with more affordable acquisition prices	Failure to achieve fixed sales goals and reduced turnover	*Putting devices on the market*		24 Financial losses < 500€	2	2
Improper estimation of maintenance costs	Veritable absence of competitive maintenance prices	Loss of market shares	*Purchase of devices by clients*	NO	24 Financial losses < 500€	2	2
Regular interruption of the application's functionalities	Server failure	Loss or modification of sensitive data to perform the therapeutic analysis	*Need to transmit health data to the health professional*	Storage on virtual servers with multiple safeguards on multiple sites Regular safeguards on multiple back-ups.	43 Complaint followed by a conviction and moderate restitution < 100000€	4	1
Regular interruption of the application's functionalities	Server failure	Loss or modification of sensitive data to perform the therapeutic analysis	*Need to transmit health data to the health professional*	Storage on virtual servers with multiple safeguards on multiple sites Regular safeguards on multiple back-ups.	34 Financial losses between 500€ and 5000€	3	1

Risk	Cause	Feared event	Use context	Safeguards	Consequence			
Absence of regular data safeguard protocols	Uncontrolled safeguard	Loss of sensitive data	*Use of the application to transmit or follow health data*	Server analysis and data reintegration if necessary. Storage on virtual servers with multiple safeguards on multiple sites. Regular safeguards on multiple back-ups.	32 Data recovery or correction with major financial losses < 1000€	3	2	1
			Remote patient care	Server analysis and data reintegration if necessary. Storage on virtual servers with multiple safeguards on multiple sites. Regular safeguards on multiple back-ups.	54 Permanent disability or death	5	1	
Loss or modification of strategic data for patient follow-up	Problem linked to the systematic safeguard protocol	Error in diagnostic, analytical, and therapeutic decisions	*Need to use the device*	Informative tables given to the client upon purchase of the device. They give explanations of: -operating instructions -measurement -safety recommendations -warnings before first use of the functions	14 Client dissatisfaction without claims	1	2	1
Partial alteration of the device's physical integrity	Device left within reach of children	Inability to take a temperature reading						
Obtention of corrupted (lost, altered) data	Injection of a malicious file	Error in diagnostic, analytical, and therapeutic decisions	*Reception and display of data by the health professional for care provision*	Server analysis and data reintegration if necessary. Storage on virtual servers with multiple safeguards on multiple sites. Regular safeguards on multiple back-ups.	43 Complaint followed by a conviction and moderate restitution < 100000€	4	1	

Obtention of corrupted (lost, altered) data	Injection of a malicious file	Error in diagnostic, analytical, and therapeutic decisions	*Reception and display of data by the health professional for care provision*	Server analysis and data reintegration if necessary. Storage on virtual servers with multiple safeguards on multiple sites. Regular safeguards on multiple back-ups.	54 Permanent disability or death	5	1	I
Inability of the patient to connect to the application	Improper input protocol after intrusion by a malicious actor	Consequent disturbance of patient care	*Need to transmit data for remote care*	Implementation of the following protocols: 1-FIREWALL that allows access to the server port to be blocked. 2- Level 7 FIREWALL that allows the presence of viruses in the software layer to be detected.	22 Data recovery or correction with minor financial losses < 500€	2	2	I
Inability of the patient to connect to the application	Improper input protocol by a malicious actor	Inability to transmit health data for care provision	*Need to transmit data for remote care*	Implementation of the following protocols: 1-FIREWALL that allows access to the server port to be blocked. 2- Level 7 FIREWALL that allows the presence of viruses in the software layer to be detected.	33 Withdrawn authorization or lockout (by the CNIL) of data + amends < 3000€	3	2	I

Total compromise of the application's server	Injection of a malicious file	Inability to make a therapeutic decision due to a lack of health data	*Need to transmit data for remote care*	Implementation of the following protocols: 1-FIREWALL that allows access to the server port to be blocked. 2- Level 7 FIREWALL that allows the presence of viruses in the software layer to be detected.	14 Client dissatisfaction without claims	1	2
Indicator management is performed by unqualified personnel	Absence of definition, implementation, and follow-up on the device's performance indicators	Obtention of unreliable data	*Remote temperature reading with the device*	Hiring of a person capable of managing this kind of procedure at the warehouse by educating the person currently in this position if necessary	34 Financial losses between 500€ and 5000€	3	1
Indicator management is performed by unqualified personnel	Absence of definition, implementation, and follow-up on the device's performance indicators	Obtention of unreliable data	*Remote temperature reading with the device*	Hiring of a person capable of managing this kind of procedure at the warehouse by educating the person currently in this position if necessary	14 Client dissatisfaction without claims	1	2
Falsification of the application's queries	Execution or intrusion of a malicious file	Third-party claims	*Free access to health data (by unauthorized people)*	Implementation of the following protocols: 1-FIREWALL that allows access to the server port to be blocked. 2- Level 7 FIREWALL that allows the presence of viruses in the software layer to be detected.	23 Orders to stop processing litigious data	2	2

Failure	Cause	Effect	Use	Existing controls	Criticality				Reference	Recommended action
Patient refusal to transmit his or her data	Absence of informed and written patient consent on data management	Cancellation of remote care	*Irritation of the health professional*	Patient excluded due to lack of signature for informed consent.	34 Financial losses between 500€ and 5000€	3	2	1		
Patient refusal to transmit his or her data	Absence of informed and written patient consent on data management	Disturbed or delayed remote care	*Irritation of the health professional*	Patient excluded due to lack of signature for informed consent.	24 Financial losses < 500€	2	2	1	A3	
Putting one or several batches of defective devices on the market	Design flaws in one or more thermometers put on the market	Clients publicize their dissatisfaction	*Use of the devices by clients*	Design qualification Product-sampling procedure at the warehouse Product recall procedure (catastrophic)	43 Complaint followed by a conviction and moderate restitution < 100000€	4	3	2		Educating personnel on (sample) quality control for products at the warehouse
Putting one or several batches of defective devices on the market	Design flaws in one or more thermometers put on the market	Clients publicize their dissatisfaction	*Use of the devices by clients*	Design qualification Product-sampling procedure at the warehouse Product recall procedure (catastrophic)	24 Financial losses < 500€	2	1		A17	Implementation of a mechanism to listen to clients, operational 24 hours a day
Complex operating instructions	Poor product demonstration to target clients	Obtention of unreliable data due to an improper choice of measurement mode	*Remote temperature reading by a client*	Informative tables given to the client upon purchase of the device. They give explanations of: -operating instructions -measurement -safety recommendations -warnings before first use of the functions	14 Client dissatisfaction without claims	1	2			

Illegal data use	Inexperienced health professional for participation in required care (assigned or in training)	Health data not registered in the patient file	*Patient care*	NO	23 Orders to stop processing litigious data	2	1	1
Illegal data use	Inexperienced health professional for participation in required care (assigned or in training)	Invalid, incomplete patient file	*Patient care*	NO	23 Orders to stop processing litigious data	2	3	1
Illegal data use	Inexperienced health professional for participation in required care (assigned or in training)	Diagnosis inconsistent with the recommendations relative to remote care [telehealth and/or telemedicine]	*Patient care*	NO	23 Orders to stop processing litigious data	2	3	1
Creation of the patient file by a replacement doctor who is unaware of telemedicine and/or telehealth	Unavailability of the health professional after a change in planning	Error or improper interpretation of the medical record	*Analysis of the patient file by the health professional*	NO	23 Orders to stop processing litigious data	2	3	1
Creation of the patient file by a replacement doctor who is unaware of telemedicine and/or telehealth	Unavailability of the health professional after a change in planning	Issuance of an ambiguous, confusing, and/or contradictory diagnosis	*Analysis of the patient file by the health professional*	NO	43 Complaint followed by a conviction and moderate restitution < 100000€	4	1	1
Complex operating instructions	Poor product demonstration to target clients	Bad interpretation of data due to a wrong choice of measurement unit	*Remote temperature reading by a visually impaired client*	Informative tables given to the client upon purchase of the device. They give explanations of: -operating instructions -measurement -safety recommendations -warnings before first use of the functions	14 Client dissatisfaction without claims	1	3	1

Risk	Cause	Effect	Triggering event	Control / Measure	Consequence				Action
Developer and client stock shortage	Poor sales forecast, delayed transport, delayed manufacturing at the factory, production time (and component supply)	Lose of clients, lose of turnover	*Orders placed by clients*	Implementation of a stock management procedure at the warehouse	14 Client dissatisfaction without claims	1	2	1	
Management of non-conformities is performed by an unauthorized person	Lack of qualified, competent personnel in the domain	Legal penalties (amends and sentences), market recall (ban on sales, updated product standards)	*Performance of an internal audit by a competent authority*	The responsible administrative and financial party performs the necessary verifications (sometimes *a posteriori*), subcontracting to an external company to verify regulatory elements	53 Conviction of the manufacturer with financial penalties between 100000€ and 300000€	5	2	2 / 1	A17 Implementing a product launch procedure with all the elements necessary for the launch A3 Educating personnel on (sample) quality control for products at the warehouse
Developer and client stock shortage	Poor sales forecast, delayed transport, delayed manufacturing at the factory, production time (and component supply)	Loss of the manufacturer's competitiveness compared to competitors	*Orders placed by clients*	Implementation of a stock management procedure at the warehouse	34 Financial losses between 500€ and 5000€	3	1	1	
Developer and client stock shortage	Poor sales forecast, delayed transport, delayed manufacturing at the factory, production time (and component supply)	Loss of the manufacturer's competitiveness compared to competitors	*Orders placed by clients*	Implementation of a stock management procedure at the warehouse	14 Client dissatisfaction without claims	1	2		
Improper estimation of guarantees (in terms of cost and life)	Veritable absence of competitive guarantee prices	Total or partial loss of stock shares	*Purchase of devices by clients*	Conformity with the applicable regulations with a minimum 2-year guarantee.	14 Client dissatisfaction without claims	1	2		
Alteration of the device's physical integrity	Device exposed to atmospheric conditions incompatible with its operating instructions	Inability to take a temperature reading	*Need to perform a remote temperature reading*	NO	51 Total unavailability of the device, failure of service	5	1	1	

Scared, frightened patient	Cognitive issues, trembling, joint pain	Health professional changes his or her mind and refuses to monitor the patient remotely	*Confirmation of the patient's consent to remote care*	Behavioral, cognitive, and nervous issues are reasons not to use connected objects and exclusion criteria in telehealth.	24 Financial losses < 500€	2	3
Scared, frightened patient	Cognitive issues, trembling, joint pain	Health professional changes his or her mind and refuses to monitor the patient remotely	*Confirmation of the patient's consent to remote care*	Behavioral, cognitive, and nervous issues are reasons not to use connected objects and exclusion criteria in telehealth.	13 Warning without formal notice followed by an offer for free regularization	1	2
Fraudulent data use	Non-anonymization of the data to be processed (by the host)	Civil and punitive sanction	*Investigation performed by competent authorities*	Implementation of the FHIR data format. C is a data format adapted to the medical domain. The sent medical data are separated from the patient's identity. Within the DB (databases), there is no direct link between the patient and his or her data. Due to this fact, it is more complicated to reassociate captured data to a patient identity or profile.	23 Orders to stop processing litigious data	2	1

Fraudulent data use	Non-anonymization of the data to be processed (by the host)	Civil and punitive sanction	*Investigation performed by competent authorities*	Implementation of the FHIR data format. C is a data format adapted to the medical domain. The transmitted medical data is separated from the patient's identity. Within the BDD, there is no direct link between the patient and his or her data. Due to this fact, it is more complicated to reassociate captured data to a patient identity or profile.	34 Financial losses between 500€ and 5000€	3	2	1
Inability of the patient to connect to the application	Improper input protocol after intrusion by a malicious actor	Inability to transmit health data for care provision	*Need to transmit data for remote care*	Implementation of the following protocols: 1-FIREWALL that allows access to the server port to be blocked. 2- Level 7 FIREWALL that allows the presence of viruses in the software layer to be detected.	14 Client dissatisfaction without claims	1	4	1
Inability of the patient to connect to the application	Improper input protocol after intrusion by a malicious actor	Inaccessible data	*Need to transmit data for remote care*	Implementation of the following protocols: 1-FIREWALL that allows access to the server port to be blocked. 2- Level 7 FIREWALL that allows the presence of viruses in the software layer to be detected.	14 Client dissatisfaction without claims	1	4	1

Cause	Source	Effect	Function	Controls	Risk			
Technology ill-adapted to the presence of external electromagnetic fields	Presence of an electric or magnetic source (television, microwave oven)	Inability to obtain reliable temperature data	Need to take a remote temperature reading with the device	NO	14 Client dissatisfaction without claims	1	5	1
Access to raw data + data modification	Use of a sniffer (probe that captures raw data in the air)	Therapeutic analysis error	Transmission of health data to the health professional	Server analysis and data reintegration if necessary. Implementation of the following protocols: 1-FIREWALL that allows access to the server port to be blocked. 2- Level 7 FIREWALL that allows the presence of viruses in the software layer to be detected.	43 Complaint followed by a conviction and moderate restitution < 100000€	4	1	1
Access to raw data + data modification	Use of a sniffer (probe that captures raw data in the air)	Analysis and therapeutic error	Transmission of health data to the health professional	Server analysis and data reintegration if necessary. Implementation of the following protocols: 1-FIREWALL that allows access to the server port to be blocked. 2- Level 7 FIREWALL that allows the presence of viruses in the software layer to be detected.	32 Data recovery or correction with major financial losses < 1000€	3	2	1
Improper processing loop	Improper logical calculation	Improper interpretation of the data	Device use	Ongoing support R&D	14 Client dissatisfaction without claims	1	5	1

Risk	Cause	Consequence	Context	Existing measures	Evaluation	Values	Action
Failure to keep the patient's sensitive data	Application access rights are less or badly protected	Voluntary disclosure of data by a malicious actor	*Electronic data transmissions for remote care provision*	Implementation of the following protocols: 1-FIREWALL that allows access to the server port to be blocked. 2- Level 7 FIREWALL that allows the presence of viruses in the software layer to be detected.	43 Complaint followed by a conviction and moderate restitution < 100000€	4 3 2 1	**A1** Drafting a protocol that allows data to be encrypted by the telephone and decrypted by the server, which alone has the key. **A14** Implementing a strong identification protocol to protect access to the database (for health professionals).
Inability to use the mobile device on the terminal	Unavailability of certain functionalities of the application	Inability to use the device and inability to feed the database for medical research	*Need to transmit data to medical research centers*	NO	14 Client dissatisfaction without claims	1 3 1	
Presence of reddish rust on the device	Oxidation of the device or components	Alteration of the temperature data's physical integrity	*Device use*	Informative tables given to the client upon purchase of the device. They give explanations of: -operating instructions -measurement -safety recommendations -warnings before first use of the functions 2-year guarantee	14 Client dissatisfaction without claims	1 4 1	
Non-compliant devices put on the market	Tools not appropriate for the ensurance of device quality control	Financial loss, loss of brand confidence and credibility	*Purchase + use of devices*	Design qualification in accordance with good medical device manufacturing practices at the factory Product sampling procedure at warehouse	53 Conviction of the manufacturer with financial penalties between 100000€ and 300000€	5 2 2 1	**A3** Educating personnel on (sample) quality control for products at the warehouse.

Risk	Cause	Scenario	Existing measures	Consequence				Recommendation
Complex operating instructions / Poor product demonstration to target clients	Obtention of unreliable data due to an improper choice of measurement mode	*Remote temperature reading by a client*	Informative tables given to the client upon purchase of the device. They give explanations of: -operating instructions -measurement -safety recommendations -warnings before first use of the functions / 12 Recovery or correction of data without operational inconvenience or financial losses	1	4	1		A13 Promoting the education of pharmacists or health professionals concerning telehealth and/or telemedicine
Creation of the patient file by a replacement doctor who is unaware of telemedicine and/or telehealth	Unavailability of the health professional following a change in planning or sick leave	Inability to meet the health professional and exacerbation of patient's state of health	*Patient's need to meet the health professional to verify the prescriptions made by a replacement doctor* NO / 54 Permanent disability or death	5	2	2		A17 Implementation of a mechanism to listen to clients, operational 24 hours a day
Creation of the patient file by a replacement doctor who is unaware of telemedicine	Unavailability of the health professional following a change in planning or sick leave	Inability to meet the health professional and exacerbation of patient's state of health	*Patient's need to meet the health professional to verify the prescriptions made by a replacement doctor* NO / 43 Complaint followed by a conviction and moderate restitution < 100000€	4	1			
Creation of the patient file by a replacement doctor who is unaware of telemedicine and/or telehealth	Unavailability of the health professional following a change in planning or sick leave	Inability to meet the health professional and exacerbation of patient's state of health	*Patient's need to meet the health professional to verify the prescriptions made by a replacement doctor* NO / 45 Temporary disability	4	2	1		A13 Promoting the education of pharmacists or health professionals concerning telehealth and/or telemedicine

Creation of the patient file by a replacement doctor who is unaware of telemedicine and/or telehealth	Unavailability of the health professional following a change in planning or sick leave	Inability to meet the health professional and exacerbation of the patient's state of health	*Patient's need to meet the health professional to verify the prescriptions made by a replacement doctor*	NO	14 Client dissatisfaction without claims	1	4	1
Inability to make the device work	Device not fed with data	Inability to monitor temperature readings	*Need to follow his or her temperature*	Informative tables given to the client upon purchase of the device. They give explanations of: -operating instructions -measurement -safety recommendations -warnings before first use of the functions	14 Client dissatisfaction without claims	1	1	1
Damaged device	Strong electrical discharge after a power surge	Inability to use the device and inability to feed the database for research on difficult pathologies	*Need to transmit data to feed medical research centers*	NO	51 Total unavailability of the device, failure of service	5	1	1
Improper (data) transfer frequency	Inconsistent wait time	Inability to transmit measurement data	*Need to transmit temperature data to medical research centers*	Implementation of indicators like the establishment of a Bluetooth connection on the screen, which allows confirmation that the connection has been established and the data transfer performed.	14 Client dissatisfaction without claims	1	3	1

Table 12.1. *Cartography of initial and residual risks. For a color version of this table, see www.iste.co.uk/beyala/health.zip*

13

Risk-Reduction Action Forms

13.1. Risk-reduction actions

This chapter provides an inventory of all of the risk-reduction action forms. These actions can span one or several phases of the system. Their implementation will allow major risks qualified as unacceptable to tolerable under supervision to be reduced.

13.1.1. Synthesis of the risk-reduction actions

Figures 13.1 and 13.2 show that the risk-reduction actions are both protection and prevention actions: the gravity and likelihood drop.

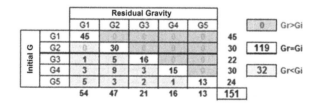

Figure 13.1. *Synthesis of the protection actions*

– Thirty-two scenarios demonstrate a reduction between the initial and residual gravity. For example, five scenarios with an initial gravity of 5 (G5) change to a residual gravity of 1 (G1).

– Twenty-eight scenarios demonstrate a reduction between the initial and residual likelihood. For example, three scenarios with a likelihood of 5 (L5) change to a likelihood of 3 (L3).

– Two hundred forty-two scenarios do not demonstrate any change in gravity and likelihood.

		Residual Likelihood					
		L1	L2	L3	L4	L5	
Initial L	L1	49	0	0	0	0	49
	L2	13	49	0	0	0	62
	L3	8	3	18	0	0	29
	L4	0	0	0	5	0	5
	L5	1	0	3	0	2	6
		71	52	21	5	2	151

0	Lr>Li
123	Lr=Li
28	Lr<Li

Figure 13.2. *Synthesis of the prevention actions*

13.1.2. *Number of risk-reduction actions per system element and danger*

Table 13.1 lists the number of risk-reduction actions per subsystem and danger.

Phase A, measuring the temperature, contains the most risk-reduction actions, with 42.30%. Phase B, visualizing the measurements on the application, contains fewer actions than phase A, with 30.76%. Phase C, sharing these measurement data with a health professional, even less, with 26.92%.

NR_FA	52	22	16	14
52	Actions	A	B	C
0	POL	0	0	0
0	ENV	0	0	0
2	INS	0	0	2
4	IMA	4	0	0
8	CLI	2	2	4
6	MAN	6	0	0
2	PRG	0	2	0
4	ETH	0	0	4
0	JUR	0	0	0
0	ECO	0	0	0
0	COMR	0	0	0
0	INFR	0	0	0
9	MAT	0	9	0
5	SI	0	3	2
2	PRJ	2	0	0
1	OPE	1	0	0
1	FH	0	0	1
6	PHYS	6	0	0
2	PROD	1	0	1

Table 13.1. *Number of actions per subsystem and danger*

13.2. List of the risk-reduction action forms

PROGRAM CRA of connected medical devices, case of connected non-contact thermometers	RISK-REDUCTION ACTION PLAN	DATE FORM NO. A1

SUBSYSTEM: Sharing these measurement data with a health professional

SYSTEM ELEMENT:
Impossible restoration, loss, modification of data

REF STUDY:
DGS/manufacturer/201X
RESPONSIBLE PARTY :
Mobile Application Manager
AUTHORITY: DG

DESCRIPTION OF THE RISK-REDUCTION ACTIONS
Drafting a protocol that allows data to be encrypted on the telephone and decrypted by the server, which alone knows the key.

If **prevention actions** → put 1   If **protection actions** → put 2   If **mixed actions** → put 3

Incidence of defining risk-reduction actions   0%   25%   50%   75%   100%

SIDE EFFECTS OF THE RISK-REDUCTION ACTIONS
Description of the side effects identified
Definitive loss of data if server destroyed
Actions to overcome the side effects
Implementing a back-up server that could take the relay in case of the unavailability of the main server
Incidence of overcoming risks from side effects   0%   25%   50%   75%   100%

PROVISIONS FOR PERFORMING, MONITORING AND VALIDATING RISK-REDUCTION ACTIONS
Performance:
- – Analyzing the need
- – Specifications
- – Preparing the computer environment
- – Creation of a program that renders the data illegible and incomprehensible for humans

Validation: Project manager
Monitoring:
- – Ensuring the introduction of the protocol
- – Performing vulnerability audits on the application

Estimated rate of the consolidated actions already performed compared to the actions described   0%   25%   50%   75%   100%

OBSERVATIONS
Reasons for not applying risk-reduction actions:
Absence of qualified personnel
Decisions made and actions proposed:
Recruitment of competent resources

Figure 13.3. *Risk-reduction action plan, reference A1*

PROGRAM	RISK-REDUCTION ACTION PLAN	DATE:
CRA of connected medical devices, case of connected non-contact thermometers		FORM NO. A2 REF STUDY:

SUBSYSTEM: Measuring the temperature (A)
SYSTEM ELEMENT: Circulation of negative opinions about the technology, spread of a serious undesirable event.

RESPONSIBLE PARTY:
Responsible SAV

AUTHORITY: DG

DESCRIPTION OF THE RISK-REDUCTION ACTIONS

Training personnel on the external level 1 SAV to be worked on together with the development team.

If **prevention actions** → put **1**   If **protection actions** → put **2**   If **mixed actions** → put **3**

Incidence of defining risk-reduction actions   0%   25%   50%   75%   100%

SIDE EFFECTS OF THE RISK-REDUCTION ACTIONS

Description of the side effects identified

Actions to overcome the side effects

Incidence of overcoming risks from side effects   0%   25%   50%   75%   100%

PROVISIONS FOR PERFORMING, MONITORING AND VALIDATING RISK-REDUCTION ACTIONS

Performance:

- Defining the personnel to be trained externally (already)
- Defining the framework (product, failure and installation scenarios, demonstrations on the device, products)
- Organizing a training slot for external personnel
- Presentation of the training supports

Validation: Indication of training seminars and proof of training

Figure 13.4. *Risk-reduction action plan, reference A2*

PROGRAM	RISK-REDUCTION ACTION PLAN	DATE:
CRA of connected medical devices, case of connected non-contact thermometers		FORM NO. A3 REF STUDY: DGS
SUBSYSTEM: Measuring the temperature (A) SYSTEM ELEMENT: Absence or improper management of nonconformities		RESPONSIBLE PARTY: Logistics Manager AUTHORITY: DG

DESCRIPTION OF THE RISK-REDUCTION ACTIONS

Training personnel on (sample) quality control for products at the warehouse (in Caen).

If prevention actions → put 1   If protection actions → put 2   If mixed actions → put 3

Incidence of defining risk-reduction actions   0%   25%   50%   75%   100%

SIDE EFFECTS OF THE RISK-REDUCTION ACTIONS

Description of the side effects identified

/

Actions to overcome the side effects

/

Incidence of overcoming risks from side effects   0%   25%   50%   75%   100%

PROVISIONS FOR PERFORMING, MONITORING AND VALIDATING RISK-REDUCTION ACTIONS

Performance:

- Defining the personnel to be trained internally

Figure 13.5. *Risk-reduction action plan, reference A3*

PROGRAM	RISK-REDUCTION ACTION	DATE:
CRA of connected medical devices,	PLAN	FORM NO. A4

CRA of connected medical devices,
case of connected non-contact
thermometers
SUBSYSTEM: Visualizing the measurements on the application (on the
telephone) (B)
SYSTEM ELEMENT:
Absence of application updates, platform unavailability
DESCRIPTION OF THE RISK-REDUCTION ACTIONS
  Making information campaign forms available to users by e-mail to notify them about critical updates.

DATE:
FORM NO. A4
REF STUDY:
RESPONSIBLE PARTY: Marketing
Manager
AUTHORITY: DG

If **prevention actions** → put 1   If **protection actions** → put 2   If **mixed actions** → put 3
Incidence of defining risk-reduction actions   0% 25% 50% 75% 100%
SIDE EFFECTS OF THE RISK-REDUCTION ACTIONS
Description of the side effects identified
/

Actions to overcome the side effects
/

Incidence of overcoming risks from side effects   0% 25% 50% 75% 100%
PROVISIONS FOR PERFORMING, MONITORING AND VALIDATING RISK-REDUCTION ACTIONS
Performance:
  – Drafting a form to provide information to users on the different dates of the updates of interest.
  – Sending out the form by e-mail.
Validation: Marketing Manager

Monitoring:
  – Indicator of sent-out forms being followed
Estimated rate of the consolidated actions already performed compared to 0% 25% 50% 75% 100%
the actions described
OBSERVATIONS
Reasons for not applying risk-reduction actions:

Decisions made and actions proposed:

Figure 13.6. *Risk-reduction action plan, reference A4*

PROGRAM	RISK-REDUCTION ACTION	DATE:

PROGRAM
CRA of connected medical devices, case of connected non-contact thermometers

RISK-REDUCTION ACTION PLAN

DATE:
FORM NO. A5
REF STUDY:
RESPONSIBLE PARTY:
Mobile Application Manager
AUTHORITY: DS

SUBSYSTEM: Sharing these measurement data with a health professional

SYSTEM ELEMENT:
Illegitimate access, identity theft, viral attack

DESCRIPTION OF THE RISK-REDUCTION ACTIONS

Drafting a protocol that allows malicious attacks to be identified in order to identify the vulnerabilities present in the software

If prevention actions ➔ put 1	If protection actions ➔ put 2		If mixed actions ➔ put 3		
Incidence of defining risk-reduction actions		0%	25%	50%	75%	100%

SIDE EFFECTS OF THE RISK-REDUCTION ACTIONS

<u>Description of the side effects identified</u>

/

<u>Actions to overcome the side effects</u>

/

Incidence of overcoming risks from side effects	0%	25%	50%	75%	100%

PROVISIONS FOR PERFORMING, MONITORING AND VALIDATING RISK-REDUCTION ACTIONS

Performance:
- Analyzing the need
- Preparing the computer environment
- Creation of a program that securely identifies malicious attacks
- Preparing the standard test
- Validation test
- Start of production

Validation: Project Manager

Monitoring:
- Ensuring the introduction of the protocol
- Performing vulnerability audits on the application

Estimated rate of the consolidated actions already performed compared to the actions described	0%	25%	50%	75%	100%

OBSERVATIONS

<u>Reasons for not applying risk-reduction actions:</u>

<u>Decisions made and actions proposed:</u>

Figure 13.7. *Risk-reduction action plan, reference A5*

PROGRAM	**RISK-REDUCTION ACTION**	DATE:

CRA of connected medical devices, case of connected non-contact thermometers

RISK-REDUCTION ACTION PLAN

DATE:

FORM NO. A6

REF STUDY:

SUBSYSTEM: Visualizing the measurements on the application (on the telephone) (B)

RESPONSIBLE PARTY:
Mobile Application Manager

SYSTEM ELEMENT:

AUTHORITY: DS

Insecure Bluetooth network, network loss or failure

DESCRIPTION OF THE RISK-REDUCTION ACTIONS

Drafting an automated database cleaning protocol.

If **prevention actions** → put 1	If **protection actions** → put 2	If **mixed actions** → put 3

Incidence of defining risk-reduction actions	0%	25%	50%	75%	100%

SIDE EFFECTS OF THE RISK-REDUCTION ACTIONS

Description of the side effects identified

Actions to overcome the side effects

Incidence of overcoming risks from side effects	0%	25%	50%	75%	100%

PROVISIONS FOR PERFORMING, MONITORING AND VALIDATING RISK-REDUCTION ACTIONS

Performance:
– Specifications
– Creating a program that allows the identification of data to be erased
– Preparing the standard test
– Validation test
– Start of production

Validation: Project Manager and Mobile Application Manager

Monitoring:
– Ensuring the introduction of the protocol
– Performing vulnerability audits on the application

Estimated rate of the consolidated actions already performed compared to the actions described	0%	25%	50%	75%	100%

OBSERVATIONS

Reasons for not applying risk-reduction actions:

Absence of qualified personnel

Decisions made and actions proposed:

/

Figure 13.8. *Risk-reduction action plan, reference A6*

PROGRAM	RISK-REDUCTION ACTION	DATE:
CRA of connected medical devices, case of connected non-contact thermometers	**PLAN**	FORM NO. A7

SUBSYSTEM: A, B and C

SYSTEM ELEMENT:

Difficulty becoming familiar with the device, anxiety, depression and pressure from stress

REF STUDY:

RESPONSIBLE PARTY: Marketing Manager

AUTHORITY: DG

DESCRIPTION OF THE RISK-REDUCTION ACTIONS

Making new quick steps available to users, taking into consideration the aspect of application use

If **prevention actions** → put 1   If **protection actions** → put 2   If **mixed actions** → put 3

Incidence of defining risk-reduction actions   0%   25%   50%   75%   100%

SIDE EFFECTS OF THE RISK-REDUCTION ACTIONS

Description of the side effects identified

/

Actions to overcome the side effects

/

Incidence of overcoming risks from side effects   0%   25%   50%   75%   100%

PROVISIONS FOR PERFORMING, MONITORING AND VALIDATING RISK-REDUCTION ACTIONS

Performance:

- Proposing the quick-step structure (content, charging, product use, downloading the application, and its use [main functionalities], illustration of technical schemata)
- Ensuring the translation of the quick step into several languages (English, French, etc.)
- Formatting the translations, rereading the whole text and sending it to be printed
- Spreading the new model to users

Validation:

- By the Manager of the technical service and the Manager of the marketing service

Monitoring:

- Client satisfaction rate

Estimated rate of the consolidated actions already performed compared to the actions described   0%   25%   50%   75%   100%

OBSERVATIONS

Reasons for not applying risk-reduction actions:

/

Decisions made and actions proposed:

/

Figure 13.9. *Risk-reduction action plan, reference A7*

PROGRAM	RISK-REDUCTION	DATE
CRA of connected medical devices, case of connected non-contact thermometers	ACTION PLAN	FORM NO. A8

SUBSYSTEM: Measuring the temperature (A)

SYSTEM ELEMENT:

Market unavailability of the devices, absence or improper management of deliveries

REF STUDY:

RESPONSIBLE PARTY:

Logistics Manager, Financing Manager

AUTHORITY: DG

DESCRIPTION OF THE RISK-REDUCTION ACTIONS

Drafting a protocol to improve the management of sales forecasts

If prevention actions → put 1   If protection actions → put 2   If mixed actions → put 3

Incidence of defining risk-reduction actions   0%   25%   50%   75%   100%

SIDE EFFECTS OF THE RISK-REDUCTION ACTIONS

Description of the side effects identified

/

Actions to overcome the side effects

/

Incidence of overcoming risks from side effects   0%   25%   50%   75%   100%

PROVISIONS FOR PERFORMING, MONITORING AND VALIDATING RISK-REDUCTION ACTIONS

Performance:

- Defining the storage location for each product
- Securing access to this location
- Defining the list of authorized people
- Implementing a form

Validation: Logistics Manager and Financing Manager

Monitoring:

- Implementing a command follow-up indicator

Estimated rate of the consolidated actions already performed compared to the actions described   0%   25%   50%   75%   100%

OBSERVATIONS

Reasons for not applying risk-reduction actions:

/

Decisions made and actions proposed:

/

Figure 13.10. *Risk-reduction action plan, reference A8*

PROGRAM	RISK-REDUCTION	DATE:
CRA of connected medical devices, case of connected non-contact thermometers	ACTION PLAN	FORM NO. A9

SUBSYSTEM: Measuring the temperature et Sharing these measurement data with a health professional

SYSTEM ELEMENT:

Straying from functional parameters

REF STUDY:

RESPONSIBLE PARTY: Production Manager

AUTHORITY: DG

DESCRIPTION OF THE RISK-REDUCTION ACTIONS

Improving the precision of the infrared wave by integrating a new probe into the device.

If **prevention actions** → put 1   If **protection actions** → put 2   If **mixed actions** → put 3

Incidence of defining risk-reduction actions   0%   25%   50%   75%   100%

SIDE EFFECTS OF THE RISK-REDUCTION ACTIONS

Description of the side effects identified

/

Actions to overcome the side effects

/

Incidence of overcoming risks from side effects   0%   25%   50%   75%   100%

PROVISIONS FOR PERFORMING, MONITORING AND VALIDATING RISK-REDUCTION ACTIONS

Performance:

- Simulating the resolution evaluation of all the detectable elements on the signal received.
- Analyzing the results gathered
- Revisiting and modifying the specifications according to the results.

Validation: Scientific Director and Production Manager

Monitoring:

- Verification of the probe's efficiency

Estimated rate of the consolidated actions already performed compared to the actions described   0%   25%   50%   75%   100%

OBSERVATIONS

Reasons for not applying risk-reduction actions:

- Lack of components on the market

Decisions made and actions proposed:

/

Figure 13.11. *Risk-reduction action plan, reference A9*

PROGRAM	RISK-REDUCTION ACTION	DATE:
CRA of connected medical devices, case of connected non-contact thermometers	PLAN	FORM NO. A10

REF STUDY:

SUBSYSTEM: Measuring the temperature   RESPONSIBLE PARTY:

SYSTEM ELEMENT: Improper treatment loop   Production Manager

AUTHORITY: DG

DESCRIPTION OF THE RISK-REDUCTION ACTIONS

Implementing an analysis system for the surface blood flow via camera/probe.

If **prevention actions → put 1**   If **protection actions → put 2**   If **mixed actions → put 3**

Incidence of defining risk-reduction actions   0%   25%   50%   75%   100%

SIDE EFFECTS OF THE RISK-REDUCTION ACTIONS

Description of the side effects identified

/

Actions to overcome the side effects

/

Incidence of overcoming risks from side effects   0%   25%   50%   75%   100%

PROVISIONS FOR PERFORMING, MONITORING AND VALIDATING RISK-REDUCTION ACTIONS

Performance:
- Simulating the blood flow density during the temperature measurement.
- Analyzing the results gathered.
- Revisiting and modifying the specifications according to the results.

Validation: Scientific Director and Production Manager

Monitoring:
Verifying the efficiency of the probe

Estimated rate of the consolidated actions already performed compared to the actions described   0%   25%   50%   75%   100%

OBSERVATIONS

Reasons for not applying risk-reduction actions:

Decisions made and actions proposed:

Figure 13.12. *Risk-reduction action plan, reference A10*

PROGRAM	RISK-REDUCTION ACTION	DATE:

PROGRAM
CRA of connected medical devices, case
of connected non-contact thermometers

**RISK-REDUCTION ACTION
PLAN**

DATE:

FORM NO. A11

REF STUDY:

DGS/manufacturer/201x

SUBSYSTEM: Measuring the temperature

SYSTEM ELEMENT: Improper processing loop

RESPONSIBLE PARTY:

Production Manager

AUTHORITY: DG

DESCRIPTION OF THE RISK-REDUCTION ACTIONS

Implementing a protocol to analyze skin composition via camera.

If **prevention actions** ➔ put 1	If **protection actions** ➔ put 2	If **mixed actions** ➔ put 3

Incidence of defining risk-reduction actions	0%	25%	50%	75%	100%

SIDE EFFECTS OF THE RISK-REDUCTION ACTIONS

Description of the side effects identified

/

Actions to overcome the side effects

/

Incidence of overcoming risks from side effects	0%	25%	50%	75%	100%

PROVISIONS FOR PERFORMING, MONITORING AND VALIDATING RISK-REDUCTION ACTIONS

Performance:

- Simulating the number, position, size, shape and intensity of the active elements in the skin during the temperature measurement with the help of programmed microprocessors.
- Analyzing the results gathered
- Revisiting, modifying the specifications according to the results.

Validation: Scientific Director and Production Manager

Monitoring:

Verification of the efficiency of the probe

Estimated rate of the consolidated actions already performed compared to the actions described	0%	25%	50%	75%	100%

OBSERVATIONS

Reasons for not applying risk-reduction actions:

Decisions made and actions proposed:

Figure 13.13. *Risk-reduction action plan, reference A11*

PROGRAM	RISK-REDUCTION ACTION	DATE:

PROGRAM
CRA of connected medical devices, case
of connected non-contact thermometers

**RISK-REDUCTION ACTION
PLAN**

DATE:
FORM NO. A12
REF STUDY:
RESPONSIBLE PARTY:
Production Manager
AUTHORITY: DG

SUBSYSTEM: Measuring the temperature
SYSTEM ELEMENT: Improper processing loop

DESCRIPTION OF THE RISK-REDUCTION ACTIONS

Evaluating the electromagnetic flow at the surface of the skin in order to improve the precision of the algorithm

If **prevention actions** → put 1   If **protection actions** → put 2   If **mixed actions** → put 3

Incidence of defining risk-reduction actions   0%   25%   50%   75%   100%

SIDE EFFECTS OF THE RISK-REDUCTION ACTIONS

Description of the side effects identified

/

Actions to overcome the side effects

/

Incidence of overcoming risks from side effects   0%   25%   50%   75%   100%

PROVISIONS FOR PERFORMING, MONITORING AND VALIDATING RISK-REDUCTION ACTIONS

Performance:
- – Analyzing the specifications.
- – Simulating the measurement of the magnetic field's intensity at the surface of the skin with the help of programmed microprocessors.
- – Analyzing the results gathered.

Validation: Scientific Director and Production Manager

Monitoring:

Verification of the efficiency of the probe in comparison to the results.

Estimated rate of the consolidated actions already performed compared to the actions   0%   25%   50%   75%   100%
described

OBSERVATIONS

Reasons for not applying risk-reduction actions:

Decisions made and actions proposed:

Figure 13.14. *Risk-reduction action plan, reference A12*

| PROGRAM | RISK-REDUCTION ACTION | DATE: 10/2015 |
| CRA of connected medical devices, case of connected non-contact thermometers | PLAN | FORM NO. A13 |

SUBSYSTEM: Measuring the temperature

SYSTEM ELEMENT: Complex operating instructions for the device

REF STUDY:

RESPONSIBLE PARTY: Production Manager

AUTHORITY: DG

DESCRIPTION OF THE RISK-REDUCTION ACTIONS

Promoting telehealth training for pharmacists or health professionals

If **prevention actions** → put 1   If **protection actions** → put 2   If **mixed actions** → put 3

Incidence of defining risk-reduction actions   0%   25%   50%   75%   100%

SIDE EFFECTS OF THE RISK-REDUCTION ACTIONS

Description of the side effects identified

/

Actions to overcome the side effects

/

Incidence of overcoming risks from side effects   0%   25%   50%   75%   100%

PROVISIONS FOR PERFORMING, MONITORING AND VALIDATING RISK-REDUCTION ACTIONS

Performance:

- Defining a telehealth training plan for pharmacists and health professionals.
- Creating a training support (paper and electronic) for pharmacists or health professionals.
- Sending the training support to health professionals and pharmacists.

Validation: Scientific Director

Monitoring:

- Demand for the appearance of the pharmacists and health professionals having received the training support.

Estimated rate of the consolidated actions already performed compared to the actions described   0%   25%   50%   75%   100%

OBSERVATIONS

/

Reasons for not applying risk-reduction actions:

/

Decisions made and actions proposed:

Figure 13.15. *Risk-reduction action plan, reference A13*

PROGRAM	RISK-REDUCTION	DATE:
CRA of connected medical devices, case of connected non-contact thermometers	ACTION PLAN	FORM NO. A14

SUBSYSTEM: Measuring the temperature

SYSTEM ELEMENT:

Failure to keep the patient's sensitive data

REF STUDY:

RESPONSIBLE PARTY:
Mobile Application Manager

AUTHORITY: DG

DESCRIPTION OF THE RISK-REDUCTION ACTIONS
Implementing a strong authentification protocol to protect access to the database (by health professionals)

If **prevention actions** → put 1   If **protection actions** → put 2   If **mixed actions** → put 3

Incidence of defining risk-reduction actions   0%   25%   **50%**   75%   100%

SIDE EFFECTS OF THE RISK-REDUCTION ACTIONS
Description of the side effects identified

/

Actions to overcome the side effects

/

Incidence of overcoming risks from side effects   0%   25%   50%   75%   100%

PROVISIONS FOR PERFORMING, MONITORING AND VALIDATING RISK-REDUCTION ACTIONS
Performance:
- Approaching the organization that manages the HPC (Health Professionals Card).[1]
- Integrating the health professionals card into the security architecture.

Validation: Mobile Application Manager and Scientific Director

Monitoring:
  ☞ Audit of the access codes' vulnerability, e.g. every 6 months.

Estimated rate of the consolidated actions already performed compared to the actions described   0%   25%   50%   75%   100%

OBSERVATIONS
Reasons for not applying risk-reduction actions:

Decisions made and actions proposed:

Figure 13.16. *Risk-reduction action plan, reference A14*

PROGRAM	RISK-REDUCTION ACTION	DATE:
CRA of connected medical devices, case of connected non-contact thermometers	PLAN	FORM NO. A15

REF STUDY:

SUBSYSTEM: Measuring the temperature   RESPONSIBLE PARTY:

SYSTEM ELEMENT: Device provider stock shortage   Production Manager

AUTHORITY: DG

DESCRIPTION OF THE RISK-REDUCTION ACTIONS

Implementing the necessary evolutions to the computer tool to improve stock management.

If **prevention actions** → put 1   If **protection actions** → put 2   If **mixed actions** → put 3

Incidence of defining risk-reduction actions   0%   25%   50%   75%   100%

SIDE EFFECTS OF THE RISK-REDUCTION ACTIONS

Description of the side effects identified

/

Actions to overcome the side effects

/

Incidence of overcoming risks from side effects   0%   25%   50%   75%   100%

PROVISIONS FOR PERFORMING, MONITORING AND VALIDATING RISK-REDUCTION ACTIONS

Performance:

- Studying the implementation (installation and performance of the tool) in the laboratory.
- Defining the personnel to be trained who will be able to use the device.
- Defining the level of training by profile and module.
- Organizing a training slot for personnel.

Validation: Information System (IS) Manager.

Monitoring:

- Defining and implementing a file follow-up indicator.

Estimated rate of the consolidated actions already performed compared to the actions described   0%   25%   50%   75%   100%

OBSERVATIONS

/

Reasons for not applying risk-reduction actions:

/

Decisions made and actions proposed:

Figure 13.17. *Risk-reduction action plan, reference A15*

PROGRAM	RISK-REDUCTION ACTION	DATE:
CRA of connected medical devices, case of connected non-contact thermometers	**PLAN**	FORM NO. A16

SUBSYSTEM: Measuring the temperature

SYSTEM ELEMENT: Device provider stock shortage

REF STUDY:

RESPONSIBLE PARTY:
Production Manager

AUTHORITY: DG

DESCRIPTION OF THE RISK-REDUCTION ACTIONS

Drafting a certificate procedure for exchanges with the POPs.

If prevention actions → put 1   If protection actions → put 2   If mixed actions → put 3

Incidence of defining risk-reduction actions   0%   25%   50%   75%   100%

SIDE EFFECTS OF THE RISK-REDUCTION ACTIONS

Description of the side effects identified

/

Actions to overcome the side effects

/

Incidence of overcoming risks from side effects   0%   25%   50%   75%   100%

PROVISIONS FOR PERFORMING, MONITORING AND VALIDATING RISK-REDUCTION ACTIONS

Performance:

- Preparing the computer environment
- Creation of a program that will allow the application's servers to be certified
- Preparing the standard test
- Validation test

Validation: Application Manager

Monitoring:

- Vulnerability audit

Estimated rate of the consolidated actions already performed compared to the actions described   0%   25%   50%   75%   100%

OBSERVATIONS

/

Reasons for not applying risk-reduction actions:

- Resource unavailability

Decisions made and actions proposed:

- Recruitment of qualified personnel

Figure 13.18. *Risk-reduction action plan, reference A16*

PROGRAM	RISK-REDUCTION ACTION	DATE:

PROGRAM
CRA of connected medical devices, case of connected non-contact thermometers

RISK-REDUCTION ACTION PLAN

DATE:
FORM NO. A17
REF STUDY:
DGS/manufacturer/201x
RESPONSIBLE PARTY:
Production Manager
AUTHORITY: DG

SUBSYSTEM: Measuring the temperature

SYSTEM ELEMENT: Absence or improper management of nonconformities

DESCRIPTION OF THE RISK-REDUCTION ACTIONS

Implementation of a product launching procedure with all the elements necessary for launch.

If **prevention actions** ➔ put 1   If **protection actions** ➔ put 2   If **mixed actions** ➔ put 3

Incidence of defining risk-reduction actions   0%   25%   50%   75%   100%

SIDE EFFECTS OF THE RISK-REDUCTION ACTIONS

Description of the side effects identified

/

Actions to overcome the side effects

/

Incidence of overcoming risks from side effects   0%   25%   50%   75%   100%

PROVISIONS FOR PERFORMING, MONITORING AND VALIDATING RISK-REDUCTION ACTIONS

Performance:
- Specifications
- Drafting the product manufacturing form
- Prototype validation test

Validation:

Monitoring:
- Monthly quality audit

Estimated rate of the consolidated actions already performed compared to the actions described   0%   25%   50%   75%   100%

OBSERVATIONS

/

Reasons for not applying risk-reduction actions:
- Unavailability of qualified resources

Decisions made and actions proposed:
- Recruitment of qualified personnel

Figure 13.19. *Risk-reduction action plan, reference A17*

13.2.1. Number of security parameters per system element and danger

Figure 13.20 lists the number of security parameters per subsystem and danger.

NR_FP⁵	5	3	2	0
5	Param	A	B	C
0	POL	0	0	0
0	ENV	0	0	0
0	INS	0	0	0
1	IMA	1	0	0
0	CLI	0	0	0
0	MAN	0	0	0
0	PRG	0	0	0
0	ETH	0	0	0
0	JUR	0	0	0
0	ECO	0	0	0
0	COMR	0	0	0
0	INFR	0	0	0
0	MAT	0	0	0
2	SI	0	2	0
0	PRJ	0	0	0
0	OPE	0	0	0
0	FH	0	0	0
2	PHYS	2	0	0
0	PROD	0	0	0

Figure 13.20. *Table of security parameters*

Phase A, measuring the body temperature, contains more security parameters than phase B, visualizing the measurements on the application (on the telephone). Phase C, sharing temperature data with a health professional, does not contain any parameter.

All the security parameters are detailed later in this chapter.

PROGRAM	SECURITY	DATE: 10/2015

PROGRAM
CRA linked to the use of the connected non-contact thermometer, connected medical device

SECURITY PARAMETERS CATALOGUE

DATE: 10/2015
PARAMETER File No. P1
ASSOCIATED ACTIONS File No.A10, A11, A12

SUBSYSTEM: Measuring the temperature

SYSTEM ELEMENT: Improper processing loop

REF STUDY:
RESPONSIBLE PARTY: Production Manager
AUTHORITY: DG

DESCRIPTION OF ACTIONS TO MONITOR RESIDUAL RISKS

Verifying the application of the protocol

If **monitoring actions** → put 1   If **insurance** → put 2   If **mixed actions** → put 3

Incidence of defining security parameter   0%   25%   50%   75%   100%

SIDE EFFECTS OF THE SECURITY PARAMETERS
Description of the side effects identified
/
Actions to overcome the side effects
/

Incidence of overcoming risks from side effects   0%   25%   50%   75%   100%

PROVISIONS FOR PERFORMING, MONITORING AND VALIDATING
Performance:
  – Monitoring 1/week the reintegration of the proposed protocol
  – Defining and implementing an indicator for following up on the application of the protocol
Validation:
  – By the Production Manager
  – Scientific Director
Monitoring:
  – Updating the follow-up indicator
  – Presenting the results to management

Incidence of advancing the performance of the security parameter   0%   25%   50%   75%   100%

OBSERVATIONS

Figure 13.21. *Security parameter, reference P1*

PROGRAM	SECURITY	DATE:
CRA linked to the use of the connected non-contact thermometer, connected medical device	**PARAMETERS** **CATALOGUE**	PARAMETER File No. P2 ASSOCIATED ACTIONS File No. A2 REF STUDY:

SUBSYSTEM: Measuring the temperature

SYSTEM ELEMENT: Improper processing loop

RESPONSIBLE PARTY: Production Manager

AUTHORITY: DG

DESCRIPTION OF ACTIONS TO MONITOR RESIDUAL RISKS

Verifying the application of procedures when placing products in storage

If monitoring actions → put 1　　　　If insurance → put 2　　　　If mixed actions → put 3

Incidence of defining security parameter	0%	25%	50%	75%	100%

SIDE EFFECTS OF THE SECURITY PARAMETERS

Description of the side effects identified

/

Actions to overcome the side effects

/

Incidence of overcoming risks from side effects	0%	25%	50%	75%	100%

PROVISIONS FOR PERFORMING, MONITORING AND VALIDATING

Performance:
- Monitoring 1/week the reintegration of the procedures proposed for production
- Defining and implementing an indicator for following up on the application of the procedures

Validation: Production Manager and Scientific Director

Monitoring:
- Updating the follow-up indicator
- Presenting the results to management

Incidence of advancing the performance of the security parameter	0%	25%	50%	75%	100%

OBSERVATIONS

/

Figure 13.22. *Security parameter, reference P2*

PROGRAM	SECURITY	DATE:
CRA linked to the use of the connected non-contact thermometer, connected medical device	PARAMETERS CATALOGUE	PARAMETER File No. P3 ASSOCIATED ACTIONS File No. A2 REF STUDY: RESPONSIBLE PARTY: Production Manager

SUBSYSTEM: Measuring the temperature

SYSTEM ELEMENT: Improper processing loop

AUTHORITY: DG

DESCRIPTION OF ACTIONS TO MONITOR RESIDUAL RISKS

Verifying the application of the procedures for putting products in storage

If monitoring actions → put 1   If insurance → put 2   If mixed actions → put 3

Incidence of defining security parameter   0%   25%   50%   75%   100%

SIDE EFFECTS OF THE SECURITY PARAMETERS
Description of the side effects identified
/

Actions to overcome the side effects
/

Incidence of overcoming risks from side effects   0%   25%   50%   75%   100%

PROVISIONS FOR PERFORMING, MONITORING AND VALIDATING
Performance:
  – Monitoring 1/week the reintegration of the procedures proposed for production
  – Defining and implementing an indicator for following up on the application of the procedures
Validation:
  – By the Production Manager
  – Scientific Director
Monitoring:
  – Updating the follow-up indicator
  – Presenting the results to management

Incidence of advancing the performance of the security parameter   0%   25%   50%   75%   100%

OBSERVATIONS
/

Figure 13.23. *Security parameter, reference P3*

Having finished this analysis of the risks linked to the use of a connected medical device, it is important to comment on the return on investments in this new market.

Today, the world contains billions of connected objects in health. Ever more companies and start-ups are throwing themselves into this new universe. It must be noted that the marketing investments are rapidly increasing. This model change and this increase in budgets and projects in the Internet of Things allows us to believe that the return on investments in this new paradigm is positive, to the point that one can decide to stop managing the risks and inform the client to avoid extreme costs.

The four kinds of actions to be implemented for the calculation of the investment return are given in Figure 13.24.

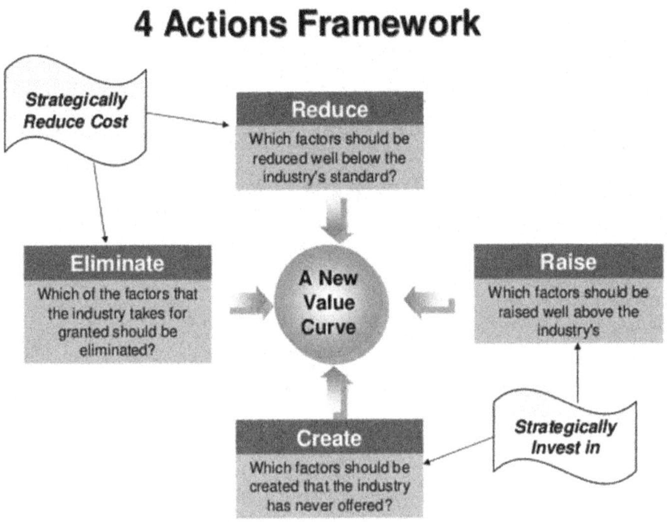

Figure 13.24.

These elements come from the Harvard "Blue Ocean Strategy" and Porter's idea of Competitive Advantage.

Conclusion

Comprehensive risk analysis is a tool and not an end. For the system studied, the objective of this process is to manage the risks linked to the use of the connected medical device to make a reliable, secure, high-quality product available to the public. To do this, we have proposed risk-reduction actions, taking into account vulnerabilities, such as the client, the image, the information system, the physicochemical and the human factor. The application of these risk management actions will be the object of monitoring and the residual risks will be kept under control. The implementation of this comprehensive analysis of the risks linked to the use of a connected medical device like a connected non-contact thermometer shows real engagement on the manufacturers' part in a risk-mastery process, which has given rise to collective awareness of the potential danger. Faced with the danger recognized, this is a pertinent strategy from the organization that quite often prevails in the field of prevention.

For the case study that we just performed, such a strategy integrates the reinforcement of the system for sharing data with third parties, the education and sensitization of actors to telemedicine, and devices to detect malicious acts.

Many of the risks found by the applications or software (of these devices) are common to the domain of m-health or telehealth. These new health approaches propose major solutions and opportunities with clinical, social and financial benefits that in no way lead us to believe that there will be any regress. The risks that are linked to this have probably not all been identified yet and it will be necessary in a later study, for example, to have a systematic approach on a multiparametric solution in which there is an aggregation of different sensors and stronger access for health professionals to the system.

The analysis of the current systems provides a glimpse into some solutions in which there are various actors (the patient, the doctor, the nurse, the pharmacist, the assistant, etc.) who all have multiple sensors as well as multiple means of communicating (smartphone, tablet, hub, directly communicating objects, etc.) and in which artificial intelligence still takes up more space.

Glossary

Accident scenario: Sequence or succession of events leading to an accident.

Connected object: "Communicating object".

To provide a simple definition of a connected object, we will define each word making up the term "connected object":

– **Object**: "Solid item considered to be a whole, fabricated by man and intended for a certain use".

– **Connect**: "Bringing together, linking things with one another. Technically, establishing an electric, hydraulic, etc., connection between various organs or machines. Establishing a connection with a computer network".

– **Communicating**: "This is said of one thing that communicates with another".

– **Communicate**: "Send something from one object to another, from one person to another".

If the four definitions above are trusted, a connected object is an item fabricated by man, whose use is to establish a link in order to send diverse and varied information to another object or to all other connected items.

Contact cause: Exposure or destabilization factor.

Cryptology: The science of secrets, this is a science that endeavors to encipher messages in order to guarantee their origin and confidentiality.

Danger: Potential for harm or damage to people, goods or the environment.

Dangerous element: Element of a system or of its environment presenting a danger.

Dangerous event: Event associated with the occurrence of a danger.

Dangerous situation: State of the system in the presence of a danger or threat.

Emissivity: Emissivity of a material (often written ε) is a dimensionless (unitless) number. It deals with a material's radiation. It is the connection between the energy radiated by a material and Planck's Law. Thus, an ideal black body has an emissivity of 1 ($\varepsilon = 1$) while any real material has an emissivity less than 1 ($\varepsilon < 1$).

Feared event: Undesirable event likely to cause harm or damage to the system according to the level of harmfulness it demonstrates.

Firewalls: This is equipment allowing the enforcement of a network security policy, defining the types of authorized communication on a particular computer network. They regulate the prevention of applications and packets.

Peering: In computer science, this is the practice of exchanging Internet traffic with peers.

People concerned: The people concerned by personal data processing are those referred to by these data that are the object of processing.

Personal health data: All information concerning an identified or identifiable physical person (person concerned); a person is considered identifiable if they can be identified, directly or indirectly, notably in reference to an identification number or to one or several specific elements, specific to their physical, physiological, psychological, economic, cultural or social identity.

Prevention (action): Action modifying the system or its exploitation to reduce the probable occurrence of an event.

Primer cause: Initiation factor for harmfulness.

Protection (action): Action modifying the system to reduce the gravity of the consequences of a feared event.

Risk: Measurement of the dangerous or accidental situation. This is a magnitude noted with two measures (l, g) associated with the occurrence of an undesirable or feared event, where g is the value of the gravity of the consequences of the feared event and l is the likelihood of the event occurring.

System: All the material, software and human elements that interact are organized to perform a given activity in given conditions (deadlines, finances, environments, etc.).

Telemedicine: Form of remote medical practice using information and communication technologies. It involves one or several health professionals, among themselves or with a patient; among these professionals, there is necessarily a medical professional and, if necessary, other professionals providing their care to the patient.

The party responsible for processing: The party responsible for processing personal data is, unless expressly designated by the legislative or regulatory provisions relevant to this treatment, the person, public authority, service or organization that determines its ends and its means.

Violation of sensitive personal information (violation of SPI): A violation of security accidentally or illicitly leading to the destruction, loss, alteration, disclosure or unauthorized access of sensitive personal information transmitted, stored or processed in some other way in relation to the provision of electronic communication services accessible to the public in the community.

Wavesoft: This is software that was developed to ensure the organization and monitoring of production costs and the management of sale stocks.

Bibliography

[BEL 14] BELLUT S., Analyse fonctionnelle externe–Analyse fonctionnelle interne, Masters course: *Gestion des risques et de la sécurité des établissements et réseaux de santé*, Ecole Centrale Paris, 2014.

[BEN 09] BENHAMOU B., "L'internet des objets: défis technologiques, économiques et politiques", *Esprit*, pp. 137–150, March 2009.

[CHA 99] CHAN KIM W., MAUBORGNE R., "Strategy, value innovation, and the knowledge economy", *Sloan Management Review*, vol. 40, no. 3, pp. 41–54, 1999.

[CHA 08] CHAMBET P., VERDIER A., "Bouygues Telecom, Obligations de protection des données personnelles et de la vie privée pour un opérateur mobile", *Proceedings of the OSSI Conference*, OSSIR, Paris, 2008.

[CHA 10] CHAN KIM W., MAUBORGNE R., *Stratégie océan bleu: Comment créer de nouveaux espaces stratégiques*, Pearson Education, London, 2010.

[CHA 12] CHALEUIL M., "La gestion des risques dans la prise en charge du patient en télémédecine", *Revue Reseaux Santé & Territoire*, June 2012.

[DER 14] DÉROSCHES A., AGUINI N., DADOUN M. et al., *La gestion des risques: Principes et pratiques*, Hermès-Lavoisier, Paris, 2014.

[DES 09] DÉROSCHES A., BAUDRIN D., DADOUN M., *L'analyse préliminaire des risques-Principes et pratiques*, Hermès-Lavoisier, Paris, 2009.

[DUM 15] DUMEZ H., MINUIELLE E., MARRAULD L., *Etat des lieux de l'innovation en santé numérique*, Fondation de L'Avenir, 2015.

[LER 10] LEROUX V., "Qualité, sécurité et continuité. Défis et bonnes pratiques", *Gestions hospitalières*, vol. 495, pp. 268–272, 2010.

[POR 85] PORTER M.E., *Competitive Advantage*, Free Press, New York, 1985.

[SCI 14] SCIEZ G., Analyse fonctionnelle, Masters course: *Gestion des risques et de la sécurité des établissements et réseaux de sante*, Ecole Centrale Paris, 2014.

[SIM 08] SIMON P., ACKER D., La place de la télémédecine dans l'organisation des soins, Report, Ministerè de la Santé et des Sports, 2008.

Documents

Commission Nationale L'Informatique et des Libertes, "Le Corps, Nouvel Objet Connecté Du Quantified Self À La M-Santé: Les Nouveaux Territoires De La Mise En Données Du Monde", Cahiers IP, Innovation & Prospective, May 2014.

Régie de l'Assurance Maladie Quebec, Code of Ethics, "Code d'éthique et de déontologie à l'intention des membres du conseil d'administration", 2017.

Ordre National des Pharmaciens, Respect de la confidentialité des données de patients dans l'usage de l'informatique, Report, 2013.

Conseil National de l'Ordre des Médecins L'Informatisation de la Santé, White Paper, 2008.

Commission Nationale de L'Informatique et des Libertés, Guide for healthcare professionals, Guide pour les professionnels de santé.

Websites Consulted

1　www.conseil-national.medecin.fr

2　http://www.itwire.com/content/view/20824/53/

3　http://www.lemonde.fr/web/imprimer_element/0,40-0@2-651865, 50-836014,0.html

4　http://www.ta-swiss.ch/a/info_perv/060506_DIV__Pervasive_computing_ brochure_e.pdf

5　http://www.unwiredview.com/2008/10/23/apple-looks-forward-to-add-rf-communications-to-everything/

6　http://www.technologyreview.com/printer_friendly_article.aspx?id=1220

7　http://www.technologyreview.com/printer_friendly_article.aspx?id=13160

8　http://www.maddyness.com/startup/2015/05/18/marche-esante/

9　http://www.journaldunet.com/ebusiness/le-net/marche-francais-des-objets-connectes-pour-la-sante-et-la-maison-0314.shtml

10 http://blog.ignilife.com/post/19251463718/mhealth-explosion

11 https://www.aruco.com/2015/04/infographie-marche-objets-connectes-wearables/

Legal texts

Article 7 of the French IETL law sets forth the principle of consent: In order to process personal data, consent must be obtained from the person concerned or one of the following conditions must be satisfied:

1. The respect of a legal obligation behooving the party responsible for the treatment.

2. Protection of the person concerned.

3. The fulfilment of a public health duty in which the person involved is the responsible party or the recipient of treatment.

4. Article 323-1 of the French legal code, resulting from law no. 88-19 January 5, 1988, the so-called "Godfrain" law. If data have been introduced, modified, or erased, the following sanctions can be imposed: 5 years imprisonment or a fine of 75,000 euros.

5. Law 1111-8 of the French Public Health Code resulting from law no. 2002-303 from March 4, 2002, pertaining to patient rights, makes the health data host responsible for obtaining a previous agreement from the Minister responsible for healthcare. Finally, health data are considered by the Data Protection Act to be sensitive and whose processing and collection are strictly prohibited on principle, unless the person concerned has provided consent.

6. French Law 78-17 of January 6, 1978, pertaining to information technology, files, and freedoms.

7. Article L162-1-7 of the French Social Security Code.

Index

Printed in the United States
By Bookmasters